RUNNING ANATOMY

Joe Puleo
Dr. Patrick Milroy

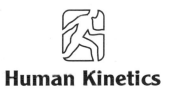

Human Kinetics

Library of Congress Cataloging-in-Publication Data

Puleo, Joe.
 Running anatomy / Joe Puleo, Patrick Milroy.
   p. cm.
 ISBN-13: 978-0-7360-8230-3 (soft cover)
 ISBN-10: 0-7360-8230-1 (soft cover)
 1. Running--Training. 2. Running--Physiological aspects.
 3. Running injuries--Prevention. 4. Sports medicine. I. Milroy, Patrick.
 II.Title.
 GV1061.5.P85 2010
 796.42--dc22

                          2009035764

 ISBN-10: 0-7360-8230-1 (print)
 ISBN-13: 978-0-7360-8230-3 (print)

This publication is written and published to provide accurate and authoritative information relevant to the subject matter presented. It is published and sold with the understanding that the author and publisher are not engaged in rendering legal, medical, or other professional services by reason of their authorship or publication of this work. If medical or other expert assistance is required, the services of a competent professional person should be sought.

Acquisitions Editor: Laurel Plotzke; **Developmental Editors:** Mandy Eastin-Allen and Cynthia McEntire; **Assistant Editor:** Laura Podeschi; **Copyeditor:** Anne Rogers; **Graphic Designer:** Fred Starbird; **Graphic Artist:** Tara Welsch; **Cover Designer:** Keith Blomberg; **Photographer (for illustration references):** Neil Bernstein; **Photo Asset Manager:** Laura Fitch; **Visual Production Assistant:** Joyce Brumfield; **Art Manager:** Kelly Hendren; **Associate Art Manager:** Alan L. Wilborn; **Illustrator (cover):** Jennifer Gibas; **Illustrators (interior):** Precision Graphics and Jennifer Gibas; **Printer:** United Graphics

Human Kinetics books are available at special discounts for bulk purchase. Special editions or book excerpts can also be created to specification. For details, contact the Special Sales Manager at Human Kinetics.

Printed in the United States of America   10 9 8 7 6 5 4 3 2 1

The paper in this book is certified under a sustainable forestry program.

Human Kinetics
Web site: www.HumanKinetics.com

United States: Human Kinetics
P.O. Box 5076
Champaign, IL 61825-5076
800-747-4457
e-mail: humank@hkusa.com

Canada: Human Kinetics
475 Devonshire Road Unit 100
Windsor, ON N8Y 2L5
800-465-7301 (in Canada only)
e-mail: info@hkcanada.com

Europe: Human Kinetics
107 Bradford Road
Stanningley
Leeds LS28 6AT, United Kingdom
+44 (0) 113 255 5665
e-mail: hk@hkeurope.com

Australia: Human Kinetics
57A Price Avenue
Lower Mitcham, South Australia 5062
08 8372 0999
e-mail: info@hkaustralia.com

New Zealand: Human Kinetics
P.O. Box 80
Torrens Park, South Australia 5062
0800 222 062
e-mail: info@hknewzealand.com

E4782

RUNNING ANATOMY

CONTENTS

PREFACE

Beginning with a chapter on the evolution of the human runner, *Running Anatomy* endeavors to educate runners about how and why their bodies work as they do during the movements of running. *Running Anatomy* explains not only how the soft tissues and bones interact to produce movement, but why they do so and what you can do to maximize your own personal running goals. By detailing the mechanisms of movement through illustrations, we hope to show, in a simple format, what happens when your body engages in running.

The goal of this book is threefold. First, the illustrations in this book are meant to aid the runner in understanding the anatomy impacted when the runner is in motion. By calling out the anatomy associated with the running motion, we hope to further the runner's understanding of how bones, organs, muscles, ligaments, and tendons work to move the body. The anatomical illustrations that accompany the exercises are color-coded to indicate the primary and secondary muscles and connective tissues featured in each exercise and running-specific movement.

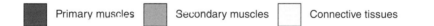

Then, after detailing the hows and whys of running, we focus on the significance of strengthening your body through strength training devised for performance enhancement. The text in each chapter further explains the function of the anatomy shown in the illustrations.

Finally, the strengthening exercises included in each chapter will improve running performance and help to keep the runner injury-free by eliminating anatomical imbalances that often occur naturally but are exacerbated by the muscular–skeletal demands of running.

The ultimate goal is to create a strength-training program that is logical and easy-to-use but also effective in improving running performance. Since injuries often occur as a result of repetitive movement, understanding how and why the body moves may be a simple way to enhance performance and prevent injury. Our intent is to enhance your running experience and performance by helping you understand the anatomy of running and develop a clearly defined strength-training program.

ACKNOWLEDGMENTS

Many people contributed to this book in many different ways. Jack Kraynak, Jay Carlin, Rob Weinmann, Dale Luy, Ken Deangelo, and Bill Preston were my coaches and mentors. Bob Kirkner, Dr. Carolyn Peel, Bill Bender, Scott Conary, Dave Salmon, Cassy Bradley, Abby Dean, Jay Johns, Sean Mick, Patty Deroian, Terry Luzader, Dave Welsh, Chris Ganter, Suzanne Dorrell, Sharon Smith, Jay Friedman, Mike Fox, Travis Stewart, Frank Iwanicki, and Robin England were training partners and guinea pigs. Capt. David Litkenhus, Lt. Col. Steven Peterson, Dr. Gregory Ng, Brian Walton, Harvey Newton, Brandon Risser, Myrna Marcus, Bob Gamberg, Bob Schwelm, Todd Williams, Dave Shelburne, Paul Slaymaker, Steve Dinote, Graig White, the members and staff of the Rutgers University–Camden track and field team, and the Haddonfield Running Company provided professional support and friendship. Models Brandee Neiderhofer, Jon Salamon, Lyndi Puleo, Anthony Witter, and Jorge Ramos gave their time and talents to make the illustrations possible. The Spa Fitness Center in Pennsuaken, New Jersey, and owner Tom Loperfido allowed us to shoot the reference photos. The staff at Human Kinetics—Laurel Plotzke, Leigh Keylock, Mandy Eastin-Allen, Laura Podeschi, Neil Bernstein, Jen Gibas, and Cynthia McEntire—guided the publication process.

Special thanks to my wife, Lyndi, and children, Gabe, Anna, and Sophia, for sharing me with this project for the past two years. Also, my efforts are in honor of my grandfather Joseph A. Puleo, Sr., and my father, Joseph A. Puleo, Jr.

Joe Puleo

My writing skills were developed through the advice of various editors of *Runners World* (UK), for whom I was medical adviser for 25 years, and the help and encouragement of the staff at Human Kinetics, without whom this project would never have got off the ground.

I could not have completed this project without the love and understanding of my wife, Clare, and the support of my family and friends, many from the running world.

Dr. Patrick Milroy

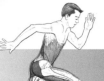

THE EVOLUTION OF THE HUMAN RUNNER

Haile Gebrselassie once said, "Without running there is no life." The sheer joy expressed by Gebrselassie about his running is shared by millions around the globe. It surpasses language and cultural barriers, so a stranger abroad can invariably change into shorts and running shoes, find a trail, and meet kindred spirits enjoying life with the same enthusiasm. Running ranks highly among ways of combining pleasure with health promotion. As civilization has progressed, the need for people to run for survival has been tempered by the development of new skills so that the average human can now enjoy leisure time in a way that the majority of our ancestors would have found at the very least impractical, and quite possibly fatal. Although the ability to run was once quite literally a matter of life and death, the social development of the biped means that running has taken on a new character. It has become a conduit for the expression of human competition, of socialization, and of scientific experiment and development. It is probably the most natural form of exercise that does not involve aggressive or antisocial techniques or require expensive equipment. Any able-bodied human should be able to enjoy it.

Although the first purpose of this book is to enable you to understand the function of the anatomy of the body involved in running, the greater aim is to add training exercises and techniques that any runner can use to enhance his or her own sporting satisfaction. Running better does not necessarily involve running faster. If this book allows you to complete your runs in a more relaxed and less distressed manner than previously, and if following the exercise schedules reduces the incidence of pain and injury, then that is surely a positive gain. Not only will you be able to look back on your previous run with pleasure, but the anticipation of the next is likely to be far more positive as well.

In the past 40 years, an entire industry has developed around the sport, although the practice of running stretches back for many thousands of years. Clothing and shoes, diet and physiology, and the surfaces on which and the environment in which we run have all undergone research, experimentation, and review in this short epoch. In much the same way that the coming of the "Iron Road" of railways some 200 years ago changed the way in which we lived, so running has entered the everyday lives of millions of people and with very few exceptions has benefited the majority. Although it is impossible to completely ignore the other interlinked factors that make a runner what he or she is, this chapter traces the evolution of anatomy as it affects the runner, researches the characteristics and physique that produce success, and even tries to predict the makeup of the perfect runner, if such an individual could ever exist. In the past, many learned authors have speculated on the ultimate running performance, only to find it bettered. We would like to envisage the makeup of the athlete who could produce that unbreakable record, and then in the subsequent chapters guide you toward making and breaking that goal.

Evolution of Running

The running skills of humans evolved as a response to predators who also vied with humans for sustenance. This was before our brains developed and we were able to think our way out of trouble. Those who could run the fastest not only got to the food first and had the biggest and most nutritious portions, but also were able to leave the quickest if danger appeared. Those who were unable to run were invariably the first to fall by the wayside because of an inability to obtain sufficient food, or because they lacked time to eat it, or because they fell victim to predators as a result of their lack of mobility.

It might be interesting to conjecture how fast our predecessors would have been able to run if they had not developed their brains and learned more cunning ways to avoid danger. However, the concurrent use of brain skills to manufacture weapons with which to hunt meant that our forebears had to rely less on pure speed for survival, and the ability to run flat out became less of a necessity and more of a virtue. The communities in those times were largely tribal, and chiefs had skills over and above the majority, so the ability to run fast would figure strongly as he or she sought respect, much of which could be gained through competition, which could include running races. Eventually, the survivors passed on the genetic makeup that produced speedy legs to their offspring, and because the need to be able to run at speed was still required, faster runners continued to evolve. In those times, pure upper-body strength was generally needed more than litheness, so those peoples for whom running had become a less important element of their life skills would probably not have looked much like competitive runners as we see them today (figure 1.1). These were people who spent their lives in physical endeavor, so they probably had a physique equivalent to the modern gym attendee, who regularly works out on a broad program of exercises but avoids specific sport-related repetition.

At some time, running evolved to have other uses. Although horses were the principal carriers of messages, sometimes people could be more efficient. Some 2,500 years ago, Pheidippides ran from Marathon to Athens to deliver news of victory in battle against the invading Persian army, though he did little to promote it as a leisure activity, dropping dead as he finished the run. Today, people and horses have an annual organized race in Wales to test the theory about which is the faster species. These early civilizations were able to enjoy sports, and one development was the organized Olympic Games, which honored the Greek gods and included running races over various distances. They lasted until AD 394 but were eventually banned because of their pagan origins.

Until relatively recent times, women did not run anywhere near as much as men, partly because they were not participating in the same kinds of foraging and defense activities; rather, they were expected to produce children, usually the more the better and one after another. Time was then used to feed and

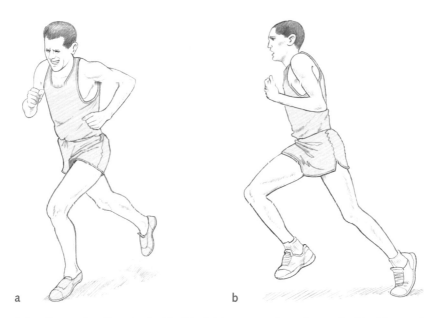

Figure 1.1   Comparing the physical build of *(a)* a runner from the past with *(b)* a contemporary runner.

teach these offspring the basic skills needed for survival until the mature males took over for the more advanced tutoring. The ability to run might still have been necessary to avoid danger, although advances in methods of transportation would have lessened the need even for this.

Hard evidence of both competitive and noncompetitive running between Roman times and the Middle Ages is hard to come by. It may well have happened, but it was not recorded by the scribes of the time who had far more important items to chronicle, so it has become lost in the mists of history. Once they had established the basics for living, people from those times were more concerned with territorial gain and religion than events that would have done little to enhance their lives. If any time was given to leisure pursuit, running would have had to compete with throwing and wrestling events, weapon skills, and the inevitable drinking competitions, among many others.

Some 14th-century texts contain references to running races held across open country, and there is evidence to suggest that competition developed from games based on hunting. In the 18th century, a new sport had emerged in which two or more horse riders would race each other to a distant church steeple. By the 19th century, simple foot races called steeplechases were organized along the same lines. These races were promoted further by the fee-paying schools and universities in the United Kingdom, who also ran "paper chases" in which a "hare" would leave a trail of paper for the "hounds" to follow. This led to the formation of the amateur Harrier Clubs for road and cross-country running that still exist today. Once again women played no part in this social convention, decreeing that it was inappropriate and demeaning to the upper classes, and the poorer majority were far too busy simply trying to survive.

During the second half of the 18th century, walking competitions between gentlemen's servants gave way to men racing against time over longer distances. One of the more popular goals involved covering at least 100 miles in less than 24 hours. Those who achieve this are still called centurions in a flashback to Roman times. Other contests involved covering one mile in each of 1,000 successive hours. (This is more than 40 straight days!) The early 19th century saw the return of races between men, and town-to-town events, accompanied by heavy gambling, for a while became the most popular sport in England.

The winners of these races were those who adapted to the generally horrific environmental circumstances and lack of nutritional variety that existed at the time. Disease was rife, life expectancy was short, and diet relied in the main on whatever seasonal local supplies were available. Any training for the events as recognized in the 21st century was nonexistent, and the pedestrians would consume large quantities of meat, often raw, and alcohol, frequently in large quantities, before and during competition. In fact, training specifically for a race was considered to hinder performance because it might exhaust their energies. It was not that they were unfit, as the competitors invariably came from the laboring masses for whom a 12-hour day of physical toil was the norm, rather than from the much smaller ranks of those with sedentary jobs.

The establishment of the modern Olympic Games was of little interest to the majority of the world's population, who had no means of entering or enjoying competition, even if they knew of it; until well into the 20th century, the Games remained the prerogative of the rich and otherwise idle, who disdained most preparation for the events. Some pioneers such as Paavo Nurmi and Hannes Kolehmainen put thought into how their racing performances could be improved and utilized the most basic sport science, but it was only in the second half of the 20th century that disciplines that could be recognized as scientific were applied to running, such as those done by Arthur Lydiard. Lydiard was different: He trained alongside his protégés, asking them to do no more or fewer miles than he, and led them through a regime that intrigued the world. It was LSD—long slow distance—for everyone. Percy Cerutty used new techniques including sandhill running to win his students Olympic gold medals.

Running and science have had a symbiotic relationship because runners have become unintentional guinea pigs for physiological testing. When statistics have demonstrated that runners have veered away from some expected normal values, scientists have been able to use the results to explain the physiology of the heart, circulation, lungs, and other organs. Extrapolation of the findings has led to progress in many medical specialities. Intertwined with this have been the advances in dietary knowledge. In basic terms it might prevent a runner from the consequences of eating a large meal before exercise, and at its most sophisticated, elite athletes often have an integral dietary program prepared as part of a whole season of competition. Medicine could never have developed to the extent it has without the participation of the running community any more than runners could have become faster without sport science.

Running hit the headlines as a leisure activity for the general populace only after the mass publicity and television coverage that accompanied the New York and London marathons in the late 1970s. In these races there was a large number of newcomers to the sport in which the emphasis on speed was replaced by jogging at little more than walking pace. It would be an exaggeration to call the majority of them competitors. This development was not only tolerated but also even encouraged as the races became a mixture between the opportunity to raise money for charitable causes and fancy dress competitions.

In terms of speed, the successful runners were those who had prepared themselves best both physically and mentally. It was noted that faster runners rarely carried excess weight, and the perception of running as a health benefit grew as parallel advances in science demonstrated that obese and sedentary people had a lower life expectancy. Race winners had usually run many miles in training before competition, although grossly excessive mileage, as in the case of British 10,000-meter world-record holder Dave Bedford, could lead to painful and career-ending injuries. It became understood that running well was not simply about quantity, but the quality of the mileage was also a decisive factor, so multiple theories of optimal training regimes abounded, none of which has yet been shown to be superior to the others in all circumstances.

Physiology of Runners

As more nations entered competition, ethnic variations in ability appeared. Afro-Caribbean athletes showed themselves to be the preeminent sprinters, whereas those from higher altitudes became the fastest endurance athletes, their bodies having adapted to a decreased oxygen concentration in inhaled air. The act of sprinting fast uses nearly all the muscles of the body during the event. A still photograph of the top exponents at full speed will show taut neck muscles and bulging eyeballs, not exactly the first areas to be considered when running! But if these muscles, in whatever small way, are used to increase speed, then these muscles must be trained for the event in exactly the same way as the massive thighs that provide the explosive power and high knee lift more usually associated with sprinting. Conversely, the best long-distance runners became almost pitifully thin, especially in the largely underused upper limbs, as it was realized that the less weight that they carried, the less energy would be expended in moving their bodies efficiently for mile after mile. However, one enemy of the distance runner is dehydration, a catalyst for both illness and injury, so adaptation to conserve and absorb water, especially in warmer climates, was at odds with the perceived need to be emaciated. Low fat stores, thin and sinewy muscles, and a low mass of other soft body tissues are not conducive to transporting large volumes of fluid internally during a run. The core temperature of the body needs to remain as close as possible to 98.6 degrees F (37 degrees C), not only to work most efficiently, but also, and more important, to survive. The energy burned when running produces heat, and it is by the mechanism of sweating that the core temperature is maintained. If the body is dehydrated, this cannot occur, so at worst a life-threatening hyperthermia may develop as the body temperature rapidly soars. This may help to explain why some winners of distance races can be comparatively well built, because they are able to store larger quantities of fluid to provide for the event. Science shows that performance deteriorates precipitously as the runner becomes overheated and dehydrated, so as with the tortoise and the hare, the winner may be the runner who has prepared best for the whole distance and not relied on pure speed to win the day.

Transposing the body types and events quickly demonstrates the impracticality of either entering the other's competition. The sprinter would quickly tire as he carried his comparatively heavy body for more than a few hundred meters, even if he could store sufficient fluid, whereas the undermuscled distance runner would immediately be at a disadvantage in an event requiring brute strength and power. These are extreme examples, but in general most events attract successful competitors who have comparatively similar physiques. It is interesting to consider how rare it is that more than one world record is held by a single competitor; where it is, the events tend to require very similar speeds and skills. Thus, Michael Johnson simultaneously held the 200- and 400-meter records, and Haile Gebrselassie the 5K and 10K, but for success at the highest level, the Olympics and world championships, very few runners enjoy the luxury of being able to prepare for, let alone win, more than one event.

Women have been latecomers to the running scene. Races for women longer than 400 meters were not introduced to the Olympic Games until 1964 because it was considered, without any scientific proof, that they might suffer some unspoken medical ailment if they were to "strain" themselves. Once it was shown that they thrived in competition, their advancement was so rapid that by 1984 they were allowed their very own marathon at the Los Angeles Olympics. Anatomically, women are generally disadvantaged compared to their male counterparts (compare figures 1.2 and 1.3), especially where the long, light levers that make up the lower limbs are concerned, but physiologically they are in some ways better prepared, especially for ultradistance running. Because they have proportionately more fat as a percentage of body weight compared to their male counterparts, they have greater reserves of energy and stored fluid to call on, although it may take days rather than hours of competition for this to emerge. It is in ultradistance racing that the performance of women comes closest to men. With increasing distance, the difference between the sexes in statistical terms in time run becomes less and less marked, so it may well be that one day a woman will win an open race purely as a result of better physiological efficiency. Women are disadvantaged by relatively short thighs, which become exaggerated by their wider hips and bring the pelvis closer to the ground, resulting in a reduction of stride length. Stride length is perhaps the factor with the most effect on the speed of running. Although the fastest runners take no more than double the number of strides of the slowest over a given unit of time, their stride length may be up to four times greater.

Although the abdomen of the male largely consists of the intestinal organs, which are involved in fluid balance and retention, that of the woman also has to accommodate the relatively bulky uterus and reproductive organs,

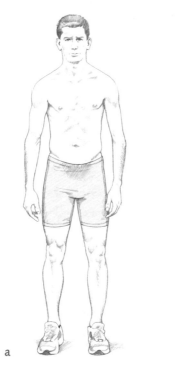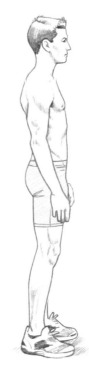

a   b

Figure 1.2 Male runner: *(a)* front view; *(b)* side view.

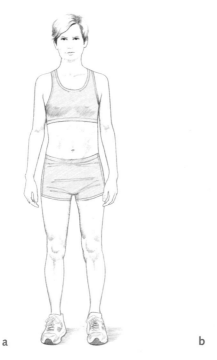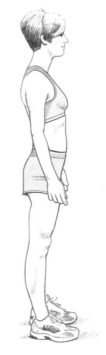

a   b

Figure 1.3 Female runner: *(a)* front view; *(b)* side view.

limiting the volume available for the bowels. These are not large differences, perhaps even only 1 percent or 2 percent, but they also determine the differences between the relative athletic performances of the two sexes. Add to that breasts and the limitation of smaller chests and lung capacity, as well as smaller feet, which mean that part of the mechanical leverage of propulsion is reduced, further handicapping women when pure speed is the consideration. However, as the male distance runners have shown, small size is not necessarily a disadvantage, and the physiological differences that become more marked in favor of women with greater time and distance run may ultimately lead to an equalization between the sexes over the longest distances.

Once the genetic core of the body has been established, there is only so much that each individual can do to develop his or her physique as a running machine. Even if one discounts artificial aids to body shaping, such as liposuction or steroid drugs, there are certain limits to the adaptation of the adult human form. No mature adult can lose or gain height voluntarily, and exercise training and dieting will only change or mature physique within the limits of capacity, such that although muscles develop as a result of exercise, there are individual limits to the amount of exercise that any single person can tolerate. So the 280-pounder, whose previous leisure activities had been purely nutritional, can expect to reduce his weight and change his shape by exercising to develop a runner's physique. However, skin has limits both to elasticity and in its ability to retract once overstretched, so the excess will remain visible however assiduously that individual maintains the training program.

The Future of Running

A problem with genetic differences is that competition can never be between physical or physiological equals. This leads inexorably to the vexing question about what aids to improved performance may be considered both legal and sporting. This book deals solely with training methods.

One factor in the improvement of running performance that is unquestionably lawful is simple leisure training. Until the last 30 or so years of the 20th century, almost all books written about running were biographies or ghosted autobiographies of the great retired runners who were hoping to make a few cents by passing on the secrets of their successes. Most of the books dealt with the races, although some had fascinating accounts of the runners' preparations—and all too often the lack of it! Although the majority of those competitors were amateurs, at least in name, the elite runners of today are as much professionals as lawyers or doctors. Running for them is a full-time occupation for which they put in hours of preparation, travel around the world to compete, and are paid regularly by sponsors and promoters for their efforts. However, the average participant in the marathon explosion of the 1980s had little desire to run as far or as fast as the Kuts, Shorters, Zatopeks, and Coes of preceding generations. Running had become a socially acceptable leisure activity, which helped to counteract the similar growth in eating away from home. Running a few pleasurable miles with some friends and then replacing the calories in an equally enjoyable fashion became the new modus vivendi.

Competition ceased to be the only goal of the runner, and running could be enjoyed for itself and the feel-good factor it produced. However, although the leisure runner became happy to commune with nature in his or her own particular fashion, it did not end all desire to improve performance, whether it be in speed or the distance covered. Running magazines began to appear on the shelves, which not only listed races and their results but also delved into nutrition, training, fluid intake and output, and all the little nuances that became part of a runner's world. The effect of running on health, medicine, and even the psychology of the sport became regular dinner-table discussion topics.

The desire to gain further health benefits and improvement from running can be advanced only if there is an understanding of the mechanism of running. Which muscles are needed in order to run, and how do they work? What part do the heart, lungs, and circulation play in this process? What are tendons, ligaments, and bursas, and why is running sometimes painful? This book sets out to answer all these questions. It also explains anatomy, the structural science dealing with all the phases of the running stride, how the muscles are employed, and the exercises that will improve strength, power, and endurance. The determined competitor also needs an appreciation of basic physiology, without which the muscles cannot function, so they may reap the full benefits of accepted science. Our hope is that by following this guide, some of today's leisure runners may become the Olympians of tomorrow.

CHAPTER 2

CARDIOVASCULAR AND CARDIORESPIRATORY COMPONENTS

Improvement in running performance hinges on many factors. Specifically, running training benefits the cardiovascular and cardiorespiratory systems, which should, in turn, lead to an improvement in running performance. However, this improvement can be curtailed by neglecting or abusing the musculoskeletal system through inappropriate training—too much mileage at too fast a pace. Even intelligent training can exacerbate muscle imbalances and anatomical shortcomings. Incorporating strength training into a holistic plan for performance enhancement makes sense on many levels. A well-designed strength program promotes running efficiency through a better, more effective gait. A well-designed running program following some simple, proven tenets or best practices improves running economy by improving cardiovascular and cardiorespiratory efficiency.

This chapter explains the general concept of running training via the cardiovascular and cardiorespiratory systems, and how positive anatomical changes can occur as a result of an educated, intelligent approach to training.

Cardiovascular and Cardiorespiratory Systems

The cardiovascular system is a circulatory blood delivery system involving the heart, blood, and blood vessels (veins and arteries). Put simply, the heart pumps blood. The blood is carried away from the heart by arteries and returned to the heart by veins (figure 2.1).

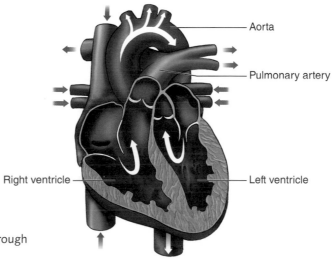

Aorta

Pulmonary artery

Right ventricle

Left ventricle

Figure 2.1 Blood flows through the chambers of the heart.

The cardiorespiratory system involves the heart and lungs. Air is inhaled by breathing through the mouth and nose. The diaphragm and other muscles push the air into the lungs, where the oxygen contained in the air becomes mixed with blood (figure 2.2). Figure 2.3 shows the muscles that work during respiration.

The interplay between the two systems works when the heart pumps blood to the lungs through the pulmonary arteries. This blood is mixed with the air (oxygen) that has been inhaled. The oxygenated blood is delivered back to the heart via the pulmonary veins. The heart's arteries then pump the blood, now complete with oxygen-rich red blood cells, to the body's muscles (figure 2.4) to promote movement—in this example, running.

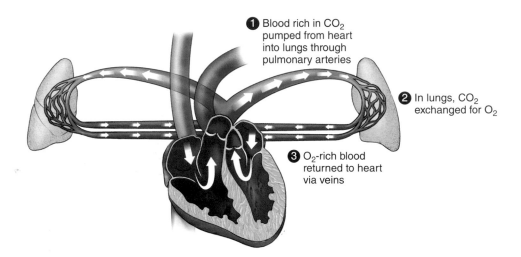

1 Blood rich in CO_2 pumped from heart into lungs through pulmonary arteries

2 In lungs, CO_2 exchanged for O_2

3 O_2-rich blood returned to heart via veins

Figure 2.2   Oxygen exchange in the lungs.

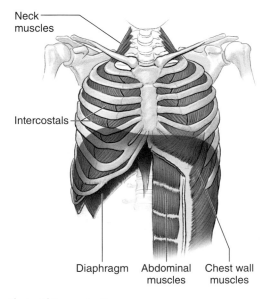

Neck muscles

Intercostals

Diaphragm   Abdominal muscles   Chest wall muscles

Figure 2.3   Muscles that aid in respiration.

How can running performance improve as a result of this interplay between the cardiovascular and cardiorespiratory systems? Simply, the more developed your cardiovascular and cardiorespiratory systems are, the more blood flow your body produces. Greater blood flow means more oxygen-rich red blood cells are available to power your muscles and more plasma is available to aid in creating energy through a process called glycolysis.

Other factors such as neuromuscular fitness, muscular endurance, strength, and flexibility are involved in improving running performance. Coupled with the strong foundation of well-developed cardiothoracic systems (the heart and lungs are located in the thorax region of the body, hence the term *cardiothorax*), these other factors will help to produce sustainable improvements in performance. The science described in the preceding paragraphs becomes exercise science, and a useful primer for improving running performance when applied to a training model. The following discussion of training is rooted in the anatomy and physiology of the cardiovascular and cardiorespiratory systems.

Performance Training Progression

Traditional training progressions consist of a well-developed base, or introductory, period consisting of easy runs of gradually increasing duration and strength training consisting of lighter weights and higher repetitions. Normally this period is followed by a slightly shorter but still significantly

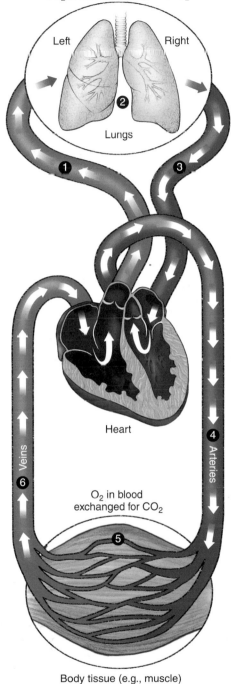

CO$_2$ in blood exchanged for O$_2$

Left   Right

❷

Lungs

❶   ❸

Heart

Veins   Arteries

❻   ❹

O$_2$ in blood exchanged for CO$_2$

❺

Body tissue (e.g., muscle)

Figure 2.4 Circulation of blood through the heart, lungs, and muscles.

lengthy duration of running strength training (threshold training and hills) and strength training incorporating increasing resistance. The final phase is defined by a brief period of high-intensity ($\dot{V}O_2$max) running coupled with a maintenance period of resistance training and planned rest (taper). The entire training progression ends with a competitive phase of racing, which seems incredibly short given the amount of time spent attaining the fitness to race. This training progression, also known as a training cycle, is then adapted based on its success or failure and race distances to be completed in the future and repeated, incorporating a well-defined rest period at the end of each cycle, for the duration of the runner's performance-based running career.

Please note that this is by no means the only concept of how running training should be structured. Ideas such as adaptive training and functional training (Gambetta's *Athletic Development,* Human Kinetics) are successful approaches to running training; however, the nuances of those training philosophies are not outlined in this book. Often, apparent differences in training philosophy boil down to simple semantics. Since training language is not codified, coaches do not always understand and apply terminology the same way. Our goal is to present an overall concept of the training progression in a simple but thorough manner without arguing the merits of different approaches.

Base, or Introductory, Training

The concept of base, or introductory, training is relatively simple, but the application is slightly more nuanced. Most coaches would agree that the pace of running during this phase is always easy and aerobic (based on the consumption of oxygen), not strenuous and anaerobic (using the oxygen present), and that the volume of training should gradually increase with down, or lesser-volume, weeks used to buffer the increase in volume, aid in recovery, and promote an adaption to a new training load. One systematic approach using a three-week training cycle incorporates four to six days of running training with a weekly increase in volume of 10 percent from week 1 to week 2; week 3 returns to the volume of the first week. For injury prevention, the weekly long run should not be more than 33 percent of the week's total volume. Two or three strength-training sessions emphasizing proper form and movement, not volume of weight, would complement this running training.

For a runner who is training for a race longer than a 10K, this phase of the training cycle is the lengthiest of a training progression because of the slower (relative to speed and muscle development) adaptations to training made by the cardiothoracic systems. Because relatively slow-paced aerobic runs take longer, they require the repeated inhalation of oxygen, the repetitive pumping of the heart, and the uninterrupted (ideally) flow of blood from the lungs to the heart and from the heart to the muscles. All of these actions aid in capillary development and improved blood flow. Increased capillary development aids both in delivering more blood to muscles and in the removal of waste products from muscles and other tissue that could impede the proper functioning of the muscles. However, these adaptations take time. The development of a distance runner may take a decade or more, while the development of faster-paced running can occur in half the time.

A training program that ignores or diminishes the importance of the base training component is a training program that ignores the tenets of exercise science. Without an extensive reliance on easy aerobic running, any performance-enhancement training program is destined for failure. A common question is how long the base period should last. This seemingly simple question does not have a simple answer, but the best reply is that the base period needs to last as long as the athlete needs to develop good running fitness and musculoskeletal strength based on his or her subjective interpretation of how easy the daily runs feel, but not so long that the athlete becomes bored or unmotivated. A good guideline for experienced runners who are training for races longer than 10K is six to eight weeks. Experienced runners training for 10K races or shorter distances need four to six weeks. For beginning runners, the base period takes longer, even making up the bulk of their first four to six months of running. Another common question is how fast the athlete should run. Short of getting a lactate threshold or stress test, which normally indicates approximately 70 to 75 percent of maximum heart rate or 70 percent of $\dot{V}O_2$max, pace charts help determine aerobic training paces based on race performances (Daniels' *Running Formula, Second Edition,* Human Kinetics). They are extremely accurate and offer explanations of how to use the data effectively.

An emphasis on base, or introductory, training does not mean that other types of training are ignored or diminished in importance. The other types of running training—tempo, lactate, threshold, steady-state, hill, and $\dot{V}O_2$max— are relegated to their specific roles in a well-designed training program. Also, neuromuscular development is needed to allow fast performances to occur. These other types of training are meant to sharpen and focus the endurance developed during the base, or introductory, phase. However, because these other types of training also strengthen the cardiovascular and cardiorespiratory systems, they play an essential role in improving performance.

The best approach to strength training during this phase is to perform multiple sets of 10 to 12 repetitions of exercises for total-body strength development. Specifically, at this stage of training, functional strength is less important than developing muscular endurance for the whole body. If this is an athlete's first strength-training progression, the proper execution of the exercise becomes paramount. If an athlete is revisiting strength training after a rest period, becoming reacquainted with the physical demands of combining a running and strength-training program should be the goal. Strength training should be performed two or three times per week; however, one day a week should be entirely free of exercise, so the other workouts need to be performed either on running days after the runs or on the other off days from running if following a four- or five-day-a-week running plan.

Threshold Training

The concept of lactate threshold (LT) often associated with tempo-based running is a conversation point for many exercise physiologists, running coaches, and runners. The science of the concept, the lexicon to describe it, and the appropriate duration and pace of the effort offer endless possibilities for debate and argument. All too often an athlete's successful performance leads to the supposition that his or her interpretation of threshold training (if it is a cornerstone of the program) is the appropriate interpretation and therefore must be copied by the masses. We do not endeavor to make any definitive statements about lactate threshold protocols. We apply the term *threshold* (please feel free to substitute *lactate threshold, anaerobic threshold, lactate turn point,* or *lactate curve*) to describe the type of running that, because of the muscle contractions inherent in faster-paced training, produces a rising blood-lactate concentration that inhibits faster running or lengthier running at the same speed (figure 2.5)—or, less scientifically, a comfortably hard effort that one could sustain for approximately 5 to 6 miles (8 to 10 km) before reaching exhaustion. It is very close to 10K race pace.

Lactate—not lactic acid—is a fuel that is used by the muscles during prolonged exercise. Lactate released from the muscle is converted in the liver to glucose, which is then used as an energy source. It had been argued for years that lactic acid (chemically not the same compound as lactate, but normally used as a synonym) was the culprit when discussing performance-limiting chemical by-products caused by intense physical effort. Instead, rather than cause fatigue, lactate can actually help to delay a possible lowering of blood glucose concentration, and ultimately can aid performance.

Threshold training also aids running performance because it provides a greater stimulus to the cardiothoracic systems than basic aerobic or recovery runs, and it does so without a correspondingly high impact on the musculoskeletal system because of its shorter duration. By running at a comfortably hard effort for 15 to 50 minutes (depending on your goal race and timing of the effort in your training program), you can accelerate the rate at which your cardiothoracic systems develop. Tempo runs, which are often referred to interchangeably with lactate threshold runs, cruise intervals, and steady-state runs, which are slightly slower than tempos, are types of threshold workouts, just at slightly different paces and durations. Ultimately, the objective of a lactate-type run, a measurement of 4 mmol of lactate if blood was drawn at points during the run, would be accomplished performing these runs instead of an easy aerobic run, which would produce almost no lactate.

A good resource on tempo-type training is *Jack Daniels' Running Formula* (Human Kinetics, 2005). The author recommends paces and durations of effort based on the athlete's current fitness and race distances to be attempted. Although less stressful on the runner's body than $\dot{V}O_2$max efforts and races,

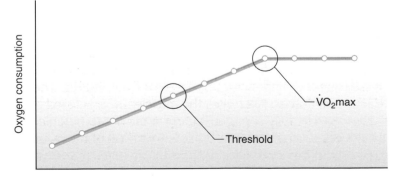

Figure 2.5　Oxygen consumption relative to exercise intensity.

threshold runs in any form (lactate threshold, tempo runs, cruise intervals, repeat miles) require longer periods of recovery than daily aerobic or recovery runs. Most nonelite runners should perform threshold-type runs no more than once a week during this phase of the training progression, and need to treat them as hard efforts. They should be preceded by an easy run plus a set of strides (faster running at 40 to 60 meters [44 to 66 yards]) the day before, and an easy or easy and long run the following day. Keep in mind that easy running still makes up the majority of this phase of training. The introduction of threshold-type training to the progression usually is the only difference from the introductory phase.

Strength training at this phase of a training progression is highly important and highly individual. The emphasis should be on countering the athlete's weakness and on functional exercises that directly correlate to running faster. For example, if a female runner lacks arm strength, an emphasis on arm exercises with lower reps (four to six) and higher weight (to exhaustion) would be called for. Also, if she was training for a 5K, functional hamstring strength would be important, so instead of performing hamstring curls, which emphasize only the hamstrings, the dumbbell Romanian deadlift and good morning exercises are more powerful exercises because they involve more of the anatomy (hamstring and glute complex) involved in the running gait. The hamstring curls should be performed in the base phase of training to develop general strength. Two strength-training workouts per week will suffice because of the intensity of the training. The muscle fibers must have a period of rest to repair themselves so they can adapt to an increasing workload.

$\dot{V}O_2$max Training

Many exercise physiologists consider $\dot{V}O_2$max and $\dot{V}O_2$max training to be the most important components of a comprehensive running program; however, this view has been challenged by some of the younger coaches who are not scientists but have had success in running and coaching. Regardless of bias, $\dot{V}O_2$max-specific workouts are a powerful training tool for improving running performance—after performing the training leading up to it.

$\dot{V}O_2$max is the peak rate of oxygen consumed during maximal or exhaustive exercise (see figure 2.5). Various tests involving exercising to exhaustion can be done to determine a $\dot{V}O_2$max score (both a raw number and an adjusted one).

Once a $\dot{V}O_2$max score is obtained, a runner can develop a training program that incorporates training at heart rate levels that equate to $\dot{V}O_2$max levels. The training efforts, or repetitions, would not necessarily end in exhaustion, although they can, but would reach the heart rate equivalent of the $\dot{V}O_2$max effort for a short period, approximately three to five minutes. The goal of this type of training is multifold. It requires the muscles incorporated to contract at such a fast pace as to be fully engaged, aiding in the neuromuscular component by placing a premium on nervous system coordination of the muscles involved in running at such a fast rate. Most important, it requires the cardiovascular and cardiorespiratory systems to work at peak efficiency to deliver oxygen-rich blood to the muscles and to remove the waste products of the glycolytic (energy-producing) process.

Training at $\dot{V}O_2$max levels is obviously a powerful training tool because of its intense recruitment of many of the body's systems. It is important to note that a $\dot{V}O_2$max training phase needs to be incorporated at the appropriate time in a training cycle for the runner to fully benefit from its application. Despite some athletes' reporting success by reversing the training progression and performing $\dot{V}O_2$max workouts at the beginning of a training cycle, the most opportune time to add $\dot{V}O_2$max training to a performance-based training plan is after a lengthy base period of easy aerobic or recovery training and a period of threshold training geared to the specific event to be completed. Rest is an important component of this phase since it aids in adaptation to the intense stimulus of the $\dot{V}O_2$max workouts. Do not be fooled into thinking that intense workouts and multiple races without rest is an intelligent training plan. It may deliver short-term success, but ultimately will lead to injury or excessive fatigue.

The strength training performed at this stage should be a set of exercises that are highly functional and specific to the event being contested and the literal strength of the runner. For example, a marathon runner who has a strong core would focus on his or her core with multiple sets of 12 reps. The exercises are equally divided between abdominal exercises and lower back exercises to ensure balance. The emphasis is on muscular endurance. A 5K runner whose focus is speed would continue with the lower-rep, higher-weight routine of the threshold phase, emphasizing the upper legs, core, and upper torso.

Results of the Training Progression Model

As in math, each training phase builds on the by-products of the completion of the preceding phase. They are not isolated blocks, but an integrated system. For example, a completed base, or introductory, phase leads to increased capillary development, resulting in more blood volume, musculoskeletal enhancement, and, theoretically, a more efficient gait. Threshold training furthers the performance of the runner by advancing the development of the cardiothoracic systems, increasing the adaptation of the musculoskeletal system through faster muscle contractions, and heightening the body's neurological response to stimulus (faster-paced running). Anaerobic training (using oxygen already present) has little practical application to distance running, and for most non-elite runners does not factor into the training progression.

When these conditions have been met, the runner can easily begin a short course of high-intensity $\dot{V}O_2$max training. The specifics of pace, duration, and rest are found in many training manuals, and the specific application of this type of training varies by individual. By following the strength-training recommendations for each phase of the running training progression, a runner is really preparing his or her body for the rigors of a goal race or races.

The result of following a training program based on the development of the cardiothoracic systems is better performance through an improved "engine" (the heart and lungs) and a stronger "chassis" through strength training. Whether $\dot{V}O_2$max is determined by the exhaustion of the heart first or the muscles first, the development of the cardiothoracic systems will permit the point of exhaustion to be reached (measured in heart rate) at a faster pace and allow a greater distance to be covered. This is a visible way that improvement in performance can be measured.

THE RUNNER IN MOTION

3

How do humans run? Is running just a faster version of walking? Is there a proper running form? Can I improve my running form? These are questions that many runners ask running experts, be they MDs, PhDs, running coaches, or fellow runners with more experience. The answers to these questions are complicated, but ultimately answerable, with a little knowledge of exercise science.

This chapter explains the hows of running. Ultimately, an explanation of the gait cycle is worthy of doctoral study by researchers studying the biomechanics of running. The overview presented here provides runners with a basic understanding of the anatomy involved, the biomechanics that engage and disengage the anatomy, and the kinesthetic results that occur from initiating the running motion. The drills included in this chapter are designed to aid the runner in perfecting the running form by fine-tuning the gait cycle.

Running Gait Cycle

Running can be understood by using an analysis of the gait cycle. Unlike walking, which is defined by having both feet simultaneously in contact with the ground during a cycle, running is characterized by having both feet *off* the ground during a cycle (a cycle is defined as the period between when one foot makes initial contact with the ground until the same foot reconnects with the ground). The two phases of the gait cycle are the stance, or support, phase and the swing phase. When one leg is in the stance phase, the other is in the swing phase.

The stance phase is marked by the foot's initial contact with the ground (foot strike), midstance through toe-off and takeoff. This phase has been measured at approximately 40 percent of the gait cycle; however, for elite distance runners and sprinters it represents considerably less of the total phase. The swing phase begins with the float, which morphs into the forward swing or swing reversal, and finishes with the landing or absorption, which begins the next cycle. In the illustration (figure 3.1), the right leg is in the stance phase (making contact with the ground), and the left leg is in the swing phase, preparing to make contact with the ground.

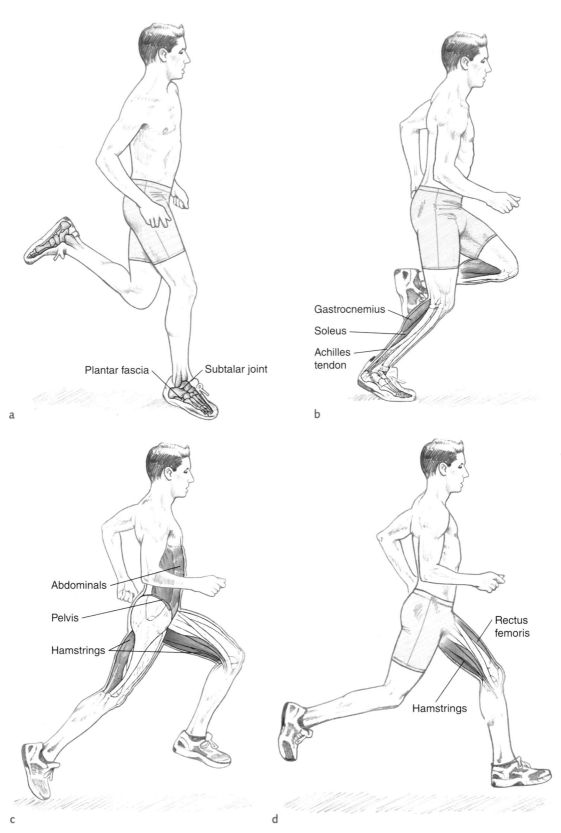

Figure 3.1 The gait cycle: *(a)* initial contact, *(b)* stance phase, *(c)* takeoff, and *(d)* forward swing phase.

Stance Phase

The quadriceps group, specifically the rectus femoris, is heavily active before initial contact. Once contact is made, the muscles, tendons, bones, and joints of the foot and lower leg function to dissipate the impact of the landing. Specifically, as described in chapter 9, three related but separate foot movements occur. The subtalar joint inverts and everts, the midfoot abducts or adducts, and the forefoot dorsiflexes and plantarflexes. Ideally, through this interaction of the anatomy of the lower leg, a small amount of *pronation,* the inward collapsing of the rear foot, occurs. This pronation helps dissipate the shock of the landing by spreading the impact over the full surface of the foot at midstance. An underpronated foot at midstance is less prepared to cushion the impact of landing because only the lateral aspect of the foot is in contact with the ground. This type of biomechanics can lead to chronically tight Achilles tendons, posterior calf strains, lateral knee pain, and iliotibial band tightness (all covered in chapter 10). Conversely, an overpronated foot at midstance can result in tibia pain, anterior calf injuries, and medial-side knee pain because of the internal rotation of the tibia. Neither extreme, a high rigid arch that underpronates or supinates or a low hypermobile arch, is ideal. Mild to moderate pronation is normal and very effective at combating impact stress.

Swing Phase

After the initial contact and midstance positioning, the hamstrings and hip flexors, the quadriceps, and the muscles of the calf (gastrocnemius and soleus) work in conjunction to allow a proper takeoff. While one leg is moving through its gait cycle, the other leg is preparing to begin a cycle of its own. Having already contacted the ground, this leg begins its forward motion as a result of the forward rotation of the pelvis and the concurrent hip flexion caused by the psoas muscles. As the leg passes through the forward swing phase, the hamstrings lengthen, limiting the forward extension of the lower leg, which had been extended by the quadriceps. The lower leg and foot begin to descend to the running surface as the torso accelerates, creating a vertical line from head to toe upon impact.

Note that two cycles, one by each leg, are happening simultaneously. As one foot takes off the ground to begin its swing phase, the other leg is preparing to begin its stance phase. The dynamic nature of the running movement makes isolating the anatomy involved difficult because, unlike in walking, potential energy (the energy stored within a physical system) and kinetic energy (the energy of a body resulting from its motion) are simultaneous. Essentially, the anatomy involved in running is constantly turned on both as agonists, muscles that are prime movers, and antagonists, muscles with opposing or stabilizing motion. In walking, the muscles are either one or the other during the gait cycle.

The role of the core during the stance phase is identical to its role in the swing phase, providing stability for the upper body, which allows the pelvis to twist and rotate in its normal manner. Because the gait cycle is defined by each leg moving through the stance or swing phase simultaneously, stabilizing the pelvis so it can function appropriately is an important task. A more lengthy discussion of the core is found in chapter 7, but suffice it to say that an unstable core could potentially lead to injury because of the gait cycle being negatively impacted.

The arms also function to stabilize and balance, but in a slightly different way. Each arm counterbalances the opposite leg, so when the right leg swings forward, the left arms swings, and vice versa. Also, the arms counterbalance each other, keeping the torso stable and in good position and ensuring that arm carriage is forward and back, not side to side in a swaying motion. Poor arm carriage ultimately costs the runner both by hindering running efficiency (stride length is shortened as a result of the legs "following" the swaying arms and rocking slightly) and running economy (poor form requires a dramatic increase in energy consumption).

Given the explanation that the gait cycle can be understood as each leg performing a cycle simultaneously, and that the same anatomy (i.e., muscles, tendons, and joints) are performing multiple functions simultaneously, it is reasonable to assume that a breakdown, or failure, in the kinetic chain is likely. This breakdown usually occurs because of inherent biomechanical imbalances that are exacerbated by the dynamic repetition of the running motion. For example, the quadriceps group and the hamstrings group are both involved in the landing phase of the gait cycle. The quadriceps group serves to extend the leg and the hamstrings limit flexion at the knee. Because the quadriceps group is dramatically stronger, the hamstrings must be able to work at their optimal capacity for the movement to be fluid. If the hamstrings group is weakened or inflexible, an imbalance exists that will ultimately lead to an injury. This is just an obvious example of the injury potential of anatomical imbalances. To counteract this scenario and others, this book offers a comprehensive strength-training regimen. The exercises are geared to complement each other by developing both the agonist and antagonist muscles as well as strengthening joints.

ABC Running Drills

Other than with strength training, how can running form and performance be improved? Because running has a neuromuscular component, running form can be improved through form drills that coordinate the movements of the involved anatomy. The drills, developed by coach Gerard Mach in the 1950s, are simple to perform and cause little impact stress to the body. Essentially, the drills, commonly referred to as the ABCs of running, isolate the phases of the gait cycle: knee lift, upper leg motion, and pushoff. By isolating each phase and slowing the movement, the drills, when properly performed, aid the runner's kinesthetic sense, promote neuromuscular response, and emphasize strength development. A properly performed drill should lead to proper running form because the former becomes the latter, just at a faster velocity. Originally these drills were designed for sprinters, but they can be used by all runners. Drills should be performed once or twice a week and can be completed in 15 minutes. Focus on proper form.

A Motion

The A motion (figure 3.2; the movement can be performed while walking or more dynamically as the A skip or A run) is propelled by the hip flexors and quadriceps. Knee flexion occurs, and the pelvis is rotated forward. The arm carriage is simple and used to balance the action of the lower body as opposed to propelling it. The arm opposite to the raised leg is bent 90 degrees at the elbow, and it swings forward and back like a pendulum, the shoulder joint acting as a fulcrum. The opposite arm is also moving simultaneously in the opposite direction. Both hands should be held loosely at the wrist joints and should not be raised above shoulder level. The emphasis is on driving down the swing leg, which initiates the knee lift of the other leg.

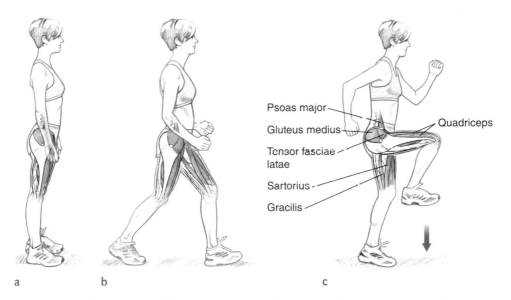

a　　　　b　　　　　　　　　　　　　　c

Figure 3.2　(a) A motion 1, (b) A motion 2, and (c) A motion 3.

B Motion

The B motion (figure 3.3) is dependent on the quadriceps to extend the leg and the hamstrings to drive the leg groundward, preparing for the impact phase. In order, the quadriceps extend the leg from the position of the A motion to potential full extension, and then the hamstrings group acts to forcefully drive the lower leg and foot to the ground. During running the tibialis anterior dorsiflexes the ankle, which positions the foot for the appropriate heel landing; however, while performing the B motion, dorsiflexion should be minimized so that the foot lands closer to midstance. This allows for less impact solely on the heel, and because the biomechanics of the foot are not involved as in running, it does not promote any forefoot injuries.

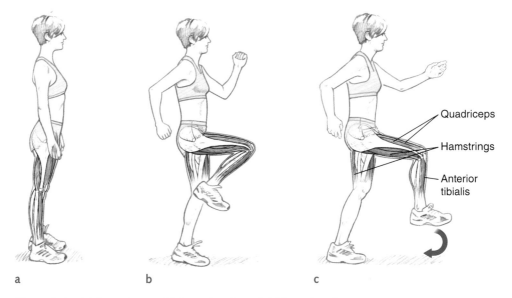

a   b   c

Figure 3.3   *(a)* B motion 1, *(b)* B motion 2, and *(c)* B motion 3.

C Motion

The final phase of the running gait cycle is dominated by the hamstrings. Upon impact, the hamstrings continue to contract, not to limit the extension of the leg but to pull the foot upward, under the glutes, to begin another cycle. The emphasis of this exercise (figure 3.4) is to pull the foot up, directly under the buttocks, shortening the arc and the length of time performing the phase so that another stride can be commenced. This exercise is performed rapidly, in staccato-like bursts. The arms are swinging quickly, mimicking the faster movement of the legs, and the hands come a little higher and closer to the body than in either the A or B motions. A more pronounced forward lean of the torso, similar to the body position while sprinting, helps to facilitate this motion.

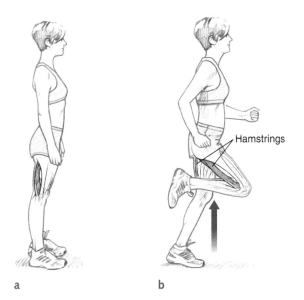

Hamstrings

a   b

Figure 3.4 (a) C motion 1, and (b) C motion 2.

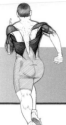

CHAPTER 4

ADAPTATIONS FOR SPEED AND TERRAIN

Every runner has a vision of the perfect run—beautiful views, a gentle, cooling breeze; a benign, perhaps slightly downhill surface; and a loving companion. Sadly, the real world is rarely like that, and we all have to make do with some sort of compromise on these fronts. The weather may be wet, windy, and cold; the surface rutted and uneven; the view industrial; and the companion a rival. In such circumstances one's body and mind have to adapt to the prevailing conditions—either that or give up completely! This chapter deals with the adaptations that can be made to cope with everything our sport throws at us. Although we have used athletes from the extreme ends of the running spectrum to illustrate the points, most runners will find a compromise somewhere between the various limits that are discussed.

Event-Specific Body Characteristics

When you attend a track and field meet, it is not too difficult to make an educated guess about the events in which most competitors will compete. The sprinters and high hurdlers are often so physically developed that they appear muscle-bound. Generally, the bodies of the 400-meter to 1,500-meter athletes become progressively less well built and smaller in stature the further the distance raced. Finally, the long-distance runners may seem unnaturally thin or even undernourished, even if their performance in a race soon belies this.

That you are able to tell roughly what type of body image fits which runner indicates that the diversity of training for an event has created structural differences in the runner. It is perhaps easiest to consider the two extremes—that of the 100-meter sprinter and the marathon runner. Not only is the latter perhaps some 10 years older, but also the years of training will have shaved most of the surplus fat from his or her torso. The sprinter may also carry minimal fat, but appears to be a much more physical presence, for not only is he or she likely to be taller, but the rib cage of the short-distance runner is covered by layers of structural muscle as well, augmented by the training program, which the marathoning counterpart lacks.

In the upper body, the arms are part of the sprinting mechanism. No one could envisage sprinting without a lot of arm action, yet for the distance runner the arms are little more than a means of balancing, to such an extent that it is not unusual to see runners who are trying to relax running with their arms dangling by their sides and only starting to use them in a finishing sprint. That said, it is quite common for runners to complain of arm pain at the end of a long race, especially if they have given no thought at all to preparation for several hours of repetitively swinging each shoulder through the few degrees of movement that has been required for the effort. That the arms are needed for balance is demonstrated clearly by the hill runner, who will invariably speed downhill with arms held quite widely open, even though this is partly to prevent injury in case of a fall.

Further differences occur in the stride length (figure 4.1). Sprinting is all about high speed. The legs can only be moved so many times a second, but anyone who can cover more ground with each stride will move further ahead of the field in an equal number of strides. The difficulty is in the repetition of the long strides, for the energy expended is far greater than that involved in taking shorter paces, which explains why sprinters do not win long-distance races. To gain the extra reach, the thighs need to be stronger, so they become bulkier and heavier, which limits their flexibility and can eventually become self-defeating if taken to extremes. Accessory muscles in the lower abdomen and pelvis also develop to help lift the thighs higher. For the same reason, the knees flex more at sprinting speed and the calves may touch the hamstring muscles when sprinters are in full flight.

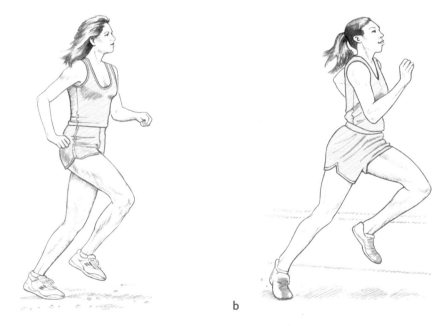

a   b

Figure 4.1   Physical adaptations to different running speeds: *(a)* shuffle; *(b)* finishing kick or sprint.

Effects of Terrain and Other External Factors

The sprinter has little to worry about underfoot. For the past 40 years the majority of tracks have been built with a rubbery surface, which aids elastic rebound after landing. These were a source of considerable injury when first introduced because of the shock of the bounce-back and the Doppler effect on the untrained muscles and Achilles tendons. Training on these tracks as they have become more numerous has helped to reduce incidence of injury. This is not the case for longer-distance runners after they leave the track. Roads themselves vary from hard concrete to soft tarmac; even standing water changes the forces produced on landing. All of these alter the shock waves and response within the lower limbs particularly. Even more difficult is the adaptation by the hill or mountain runner, who not only has to ascend and descend vertically (figure 4.2), but may also have to run slopes diagonally. This produces excessive forces not only on the lower limbs (figure 4.3), as the ankle joints need to prepare for constant inversion and eversion, but also on the knees and hips and the pelvis. The consequence of this may be a scoliotic, or twisted, lower back, which will soon become painful unless steps are taken to prepare for this type of running.

Hills are the ultimate test of the ability to stay upright while running. If the runner is unstable, he or she will soon topple over. Those blessed with a low center of gravity have a head start, although their inherently short legs may not deliver a long stride. A thin torso is a factor under the control of the runner because it may lower the center of gravity; reducing weight overall also makes

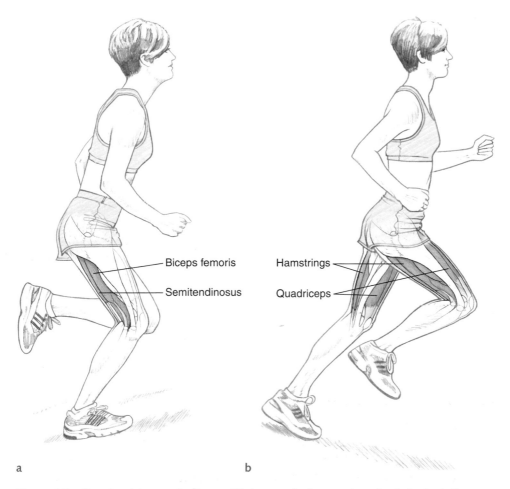

a   b

Figure 4.2 Running (a) up an incline or (b) down a decline requires physical adaptations.

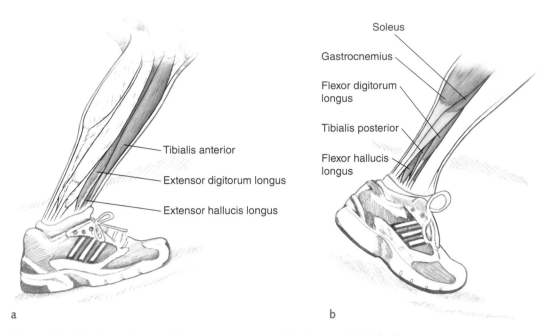

Figure 4.3   The lower legs and feet must adapt to *(a)* inclines and *(b)* declines.

it easier to lift the body vertically. Flexibility of the spine, particularly the lumbar area, is also a virtue because the climber needs to incline into the slope and the descender needs to lean backward to avoid the center of gravity from being moved forward horizontally by the running action. It follows that the hips have to be more flexible to compensate for the decreased range of motion in the spine that the need to lean causes. Although the muscles that are used to run hills are the same, the emphasis changes. The erector spinae and iliopsoas have more work to do while climbing because a tilted spine requires more effort to hold it stable than a vertical one, where the vertebrae generally just sit on top of each other. Descent places greater stresses on the anterior muscles of the calves and thighs, which have to absorb the impact of landing as well as the effect of gravity. Because running on flat surfaces cannot adequately prepare any runner for hills, some of the training should involve climbing, even if stairs alone are used. Downhill training is more difficult if the runner lives on flat terrain, although as a last resort, stepping, both up and down, can give some experience of the problems and training for hills, especially if maintained for several minutes. Climbing muscles in the calves and anterior thighs can be strengthened using the exercises in chapter 9.

Cross-country running is sufficiently global to boast its own world championships, though all too often they are run on grassy parkland surfaces. The real aficionados prefer six miles or more of deep, gluelike mud from which they have to lift their legs out with each stride while attempting not to slip backward on the treacherous ground. Although the choice of footwear may aid movement, it does little to prepare for the increasingly exhausting effort that each stride demands compared to the rebound found on the roads.

Bends and corners present their own difficulties. Runners have to lean into the corner at a right angle (figure 4.4), or they will fall flat on their sides. Indoor tracks are half the length of those outdoors and are steeply banked to allow runners to lean less obviously and be able to concentrate on staying in their own lanes as they double back through 180 degrees. Bend running stresses the lateral outer side of the lower limbs; the fasciae latac, the peroneal muscles, and the lateral ligaments of both outer knee and ankle have to take the extra force induced when turning. The medial side of the inner leg is similarly affected. Running indoors on the boards for the first time has been an awakening for many experienced runners who thought they knew it all! The shoes also have to absorb the lateral forces, so laterally rippled shoes that grip mud when running forward will give no help when the foot slides outward when a sharp corner is turned.

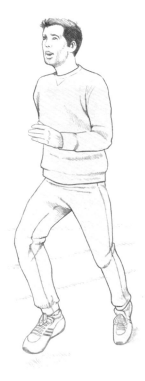

Many roads have a camber, so if a runner persists in running along one particular side of the road, he effectively gives himself a leg-length difference; that is, one leg (that nearer the middle of the road) will appear shorter than the other, and the pelvis will inevitably be tilted. In order to compensate for this,

Figure 4.4 Runners have to lean into corners on banked indoor tracks.

the pelvis has to incline so the lumbar spine corrects itself by twisting to become vertical. If a runner needed a recipe for low back pain, this is it! As we cannot recommend running down the middle of the road either, local knowledge of heavily cambered roads or alternating sides may help to reduce the problem.

For all these varied events, some training in near-competitive situations is invaluable. Although he wasn't preparing for a running event, British racewalker Don Thompson prepared for the sapping humidity and heat of Rome in July for the 1960 Olympic 50K race by steaming himself in a heavy tracksuit with kettles of boiling water in the modest bathroom of his home. The result: an unexpected gold medal. This is an extreme example that we would strongly discourage following, but in general, practicing in conditions that resemble competition is unlikely to do any serious harm, especially if adequate time is left for recovery and lessons from the experience are learned. It may not be entirely possible for runners to simulate race conditions. The domination of long-distance races by Africans in the 21st century may be partly a result of evolution, but that itself is influenced by living at altitude and by a lifestyle that demands that they may need to run 5 or 10 miles each way to school in order to be educated. If the kids in Western civilizations had to do the same, might not they have similar successes?

All training has to rely on the facilities available. A town-dwelling mountain runner is unlikely to have suitable slopes to train on at his doorstep. He or she can prepare to run at certain speeds, and may even use the stairs in a high-rise block to simulate some of the climbing action. It is more difficult to practice for a rugged, slippery, or stony surface, where a major objective is to avoid injury. It is at this point that thought about both preparation and the desired outcome is needed. If a run is likely to involve a diagonal downhill section, then the best results will come if the runner has added flexibility and strength to withstand the forces generated by the impact of landing many times on a foot that will be inverted and twisted inwardly. This stretches the ligaments on the outside of the ankle and the knee, and yet more shock is absorbed by the muscles on the outer side of the limb. Conversely, the other limb, higher up the slope, has the inner side stressed. If the runner realizes that this is going to occur, exercises to stretch and strengthen the appropriate soft tissues can and should be introduced into the training program.

The way in which the body adapts to speed and terrain can be influenced by the training program used. Many years ago some runners trained using LSD—long slow distance. Unfortunately, this only made them good at running long distances slowly and led them to other problems in the form of overuse injury. It is not only human bodies that react badly to wearisome repetition; machines are not much different and also break down with long-term continuous use. One method of prevention is to vary the programs used. As sprinters have shown, fast running is about training the whole body. Some of this means running fast, but a large proportion of the program requires neither racing shoes nor a track. It should be no different for distance runners, who should exercise specific parts as well as their whole bodies. Hills and rough and uneven surfaces can all be faced with more confidence if the body is prepared, especially if certain weaknesses are known. A cross-country runner who is aware that he or she loses ground in thick mud can perform exercises and training drills to strengthen the thigh muscles needed to haul him or her through. In each chapter of this book we have produced disciplines to cover all these eventualities, help you to adapt to the sort of running that you want or even may have to do, and aim to make you a better runner. If you are unable to adjust to the speed and terrain that you encounter during your runs, not only will the performance factor be lowered, but there is every chance that the enjoyment will disappear with it as well.

External factors must be another consideration. No one in their right mind would wear a pair of spiked shoes for a road race, but the choice of clothing and shoes for the race may well help to determine the outcome. On a warm day, well-ventilated, airy, and pale-colored attire helps to reduce heat buildup from various external and internal sources. In contrast, warm protective clothes may help reduce the greater risk of injury that colder temperatures may induce.

Although very light shoes are suitable for a short-distance race, a heavier pair may give more cushioning and protection to the lower limbs and back over a longer distance despite the weight increase. The composition of the shoe is an important factor in maximizing the value of a run. The upper parts of shoes fail to be waterproof after a heavy rainfall, though some materials will limit the ingress of water sufficiently to prevent the otherwise strong possibility of blistering and other skin conditions. The weight of the shoe should probably be in inverse proportion to the distance to be run. The grip on the ground underfoot is paramount. Spikes gain the best purchase but will ruin feet if used on tarmac or concrete, where rubber-based compounds have the most elasticity and facilitate a good rebound effect. On softer but still firm terrain, such as grass, spikes are ideal, but some runners prefer the sole to have a waffle or even a ridged effect where the ground is likely to be muddy (figure 4.5). Snow and ice present their own difficulties with the maintenance of grip. Spikes are often best, but then the runner has to beware of frostbite. Where hills and their often rocky surfaces are involved, there is debate as to which are the best shoes to provide grip for both uphill and downhill running, yet have sufficient cushioning to stop the landing at up to 10 times body weight from damaging heels and metatarsals. Experience will eventually allow the runner to decide on the most suitable shoe for any particular surface, and we discuss shoes more fully in chapter 11.

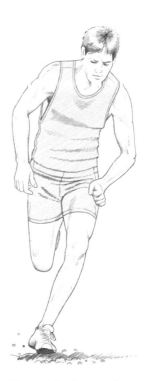

Figure 4.5   Proper shoes help a runner keep his footing on muddy or gravelly surfaces.

It is no coincidence that the fastest sprinters in the world make the majority of their appearances and all of their fastest runs in the summer months. Once the temperature drops below the mid-60s (F; high teens C), flexibility is lost in the ligaments and joints of the lower limbs and the blood flow through muscles will decrease as a result of the cooling. This is a certain recipe for injury, especially because winter preparation probably contained a large percentage of indoor training in warm clothing to simulate summer temperatures during which muscle volume and strength were built up. Sprinters require this body muscle bulk for the explosion of power needed in their events. This can only be obtained by repetitive training in muscle-friendly ambient temperatures with increasingly heavy weights and drills, which eventually produce the muscle definition so admired and effective in their events. Watching a slow-motion image of sprinters shows how they run with every muscle available. Look not only at their legs, but also watch the shoulders, arms, neck, and even the lips of a sprinter running flat out to visualize how the winner is the one who has trained each of these elements individually and hardest. Usain Bolt did not just happen!

Even if you do not have a coach with whom to discuss your objectives, there is nothing to stop you from jotting these ideas down to discuss with fellow runners. If you plan a race while on vacation, forethought about the conditions—both the weather and the terrain—could pay dividends. It could be a flat race but with one big climb up or down, or both. This will require an adaptation of your speed for that segment of the run, so acceleration during the training sessions at the appropriate point and a simulation of the hill will help your body to strengthen itself for the contest ahead. We have given you exercises to help prepare yourself for such conditions—we cannot anticipate the conditions themselves, which remain your responsibility. If you follow the ideas, your body should adapt optimally to your running needs and enable you to achieve your full potential.

CHAPTER 5

UPPER TORSO

Anyone who understands the function of a bellows or an accordion will soon grasp the anatomy of the thorax, commonly known as the chest. Bellows and accordions have evolved over many years as a way to move air under pressure and produce an air current or musical sounds. The principal bony architecture of the chest (figure 5.1) consists of 12 thoracic vertebrae, each placed one on top of another, but interlocked by ligaments and other soft tissues in such a manner that there can be move-

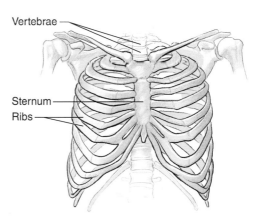

Figure 5.1 Bony structures of the torso: ribs, sternum, and vertebrae.

ment in anterior (front) and posterior (rear) directions, limited lateral (side) motion, and a degree of rotation that allows the torso to twist. Emerging from the side of every thoracic vertebra are two bony ribs that encircle the body and meet at the front, the majority of them forming the sternum, or breastbone.

Although the outside or posterior of the vertebrae are supported by the erector spinae muscles, which run the length of the spine, each rib hangs from the one above, held together by the intercostal muscles, much in the fashion of a venetian blind. Without further structural support, these would be unstable, so the trapezius, latissimus dorsi, rhomboid, teres group, shoulder stabilizers, and pectoralis major and minor (figure 5.2) all aid in the maintenance of the relative position of the ribs. At the base of this dome, with attachments to the lower ribs, lies the vast diaphragm, encircling the base of the thorax. Further stability is given by the abdominal muscles, rectus abdominis, the external oblique, and serratus anterior.

Running makes far greater demands on the body for oxygen than does sedentary life. The diaphragm uses a bellowslike action as it contracts to draw air into the lungs. At the same time, the intercostal muscles relax, only to contract strongly as expiration occurs, during which time the diaphragm relaxes and is drawn up into the thorax. Using this push–pull endeavor, the lungs fill with air and empty to maintain the oxygen needs of the runner.

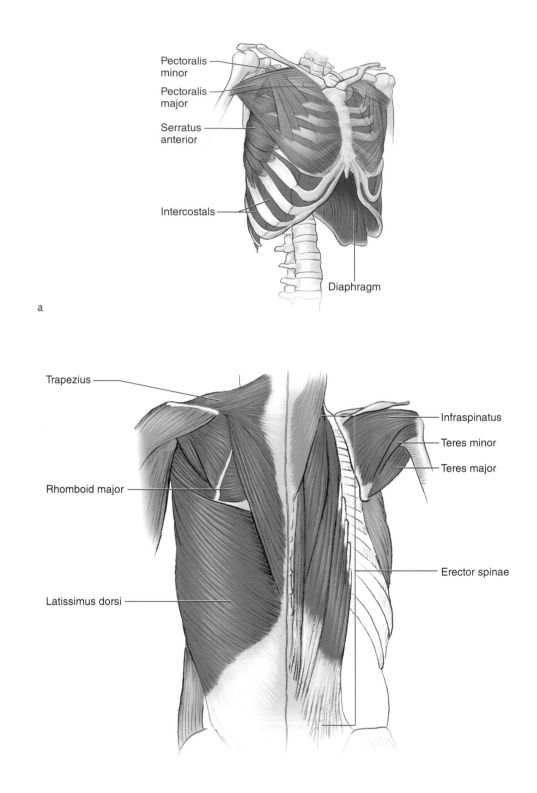

Figure 5.2 Upper torso: *(a)* front view and *(b)* back view.

As well as their action in the mechanisms of breathing, the muscles of the thorax have a limited but significant part to play in forward motion. The best way to appreciate this is to view an approaching runner in slow motion. As the thigh moves forward with each stride, the pelvis rotates slightly, first one side, and then the other. This twists the spine a little and would cause instability within the abdomen and thorax if unchecked, so a small but significant tensing and relaxation of the thoracic musculature helps not only to maintain the vertical component, but also to correct variations that are caused by forward motion of anything up to 20 miles per hour (32 k/hr).

The muscles that are attached to the shoulders and humerus, particularly the pectorals and teres, are also moved passively when the arms swing fore and aft with each stride. If they contract actively, they too will help move the upper arms to a small extent as they oppose the pull of the deltoid (figure 5.3).

The importance of these muscles in running lies with the "weakest link" presumption—that the power of the runner is dependent not on the strength that he can produce but on which facet of his running body tires first. If the muscles of the thorax are undertrained and fatigued, they will be unable to perform their functions and so reduce the efficiency of the running action and the runner himself. If the thoracic muscles lose strength and power, not only is the breathing action compromised, but also the auxiliary actions to support the spine and aid the arm movement will be weakened, leading to an inevitable slowing.

Having watched runners for many years, it is surprising how many feel that they can only improve if they increase the pace or quantity of their training. Many do not realize that the limits to their running will always be related to the weakest part of their body. The legs may be capable of a mile in under four minutes, but if the lungs do not have the capacity to provide oxygen to those legs, then they are only going to be able to achieve the speed allowed

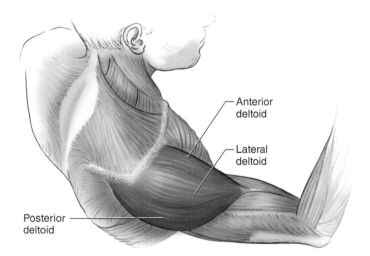

Figure 5.3 The deltoid.

by the lungs, and not that of which the legs may be capable of under other circumstances. To avoid this disparity, the diaphragm and all the supporting muscles need to be just as fit as those of the lower limbs. These muscles become fatigued by exercise in exactly the same way as do all other muscles, so it seems logical that they need to be as highly trained as any other group of muscles involved in exercise. It is for that reason that the training exercises included here should be considered as important as all those that are prescribed for the legs.

Choosing Resistance

Initially, choose weights for each exercise that provide a moderate amount of resistance but that allow for the strength-training movement to be performed by maintaining proper technique for the entire set of repetitions. The weight should be increased as strength improves and adaption becomes apparent through easier performance of the exercise; however, the weight should never be so heavy that proper technique is compromised, even on the final few repetitions of a set. Factors such as which part of the anatomy is being strengthened also factor into the decision on weight used.

For example, the pectoral muscle is large, and therefore can handle a large amount of work. The triceps, comprised of three much smaller muscles, fatigues quite quickly when it is the primary muscle group used; however, because the triceps is involved secondarily in many upper-body exercises, it will already be slightly fatigued before any triceps-specific exercises are performed. One triceps-specific exercise per strength-training session that involves the arms should suffice to strengthen the triceps sufficiently. Conversely, multiple chest exercises or many sets of the same exercise will be needed to sufficiently fatigue the larger pectoral muscle.

Repetitions

The amount of repetitions should vary based on the strength-training goal of the exercise and the objectives of the entire strength-training workout for that day. For example, two sets of 20 dumbbell presses and a set of 30 push-ups may function as an entire chest workout on a Monday, but on Friday, one set of 12 repetitions with a heavier weight than lifted Monday, followed by two sets of 10 repetitions of incline barbell presses and three sets of 15 push-ups may be what is called for. A general rule to follow is that the heavier the weight, the fewer reps performed, and vice versa.

Breathing

Exhale when forcibly moving the weight and inhale when performing the negative movement or resisting the weight. When generating movement, exhale; when resisting movement, inhale. The speed of each exercise should be as fluid and controlled as possible and should be in relationship to the breathing pattern. An accepted breathing pattern is four seconds for the resistance (inhalation phase) and two seconds for the movement (exhalation phase).

Schedule

A varied resistance-training routine works best. The concept of work plus rest equals adaption has a caveat. The work must change over time both in quantity of work (amount of resistance) and in quality of work (type of exercise) to ensure continued strength gains. For each segment of the body examined in this book, we have provided multiple exercises, some with variations, that can be used to create a multitude of different strength-training sessions all geared toward strengthening the anatomy that is most involved in running. By changing exercises, the number of sets and repetitions, and the exercise order, runners can tailor their strength-training sessions to meet their fitness needs and time constraints. No workout need be longer than 30 minutes, and two to three sessions per week can dramatically enhance a runner's performance by strengthening the specific anatomy used during run training and racing. We are not suggesting that just lifting weights will make you a better runner. We are suggesting that through proper strength training, your anatomy will be strengthened, and this resultant strength will aid running performance by eliminating muscle imbalances that impede the gait cycle, help in respiration, and help eliminate injuries that result from muscle imbalances.

Dumbbell Press

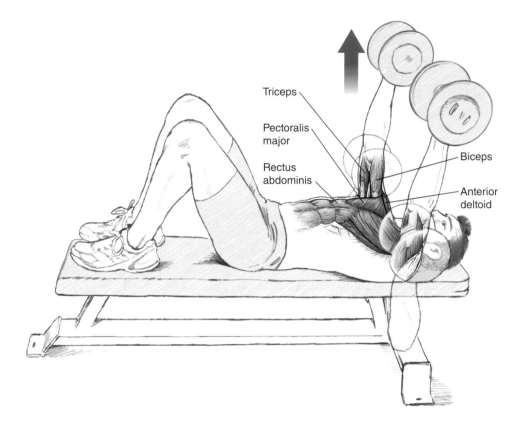

Execution

1. Lie supine (back down) on a bench with legs steepled and feet on the bench. There should be a small, natural bend in the lower back so it does not touch the bench. A dumbbell should be held in each hand, at chest level.

2. Press the dumbbells upward to full extension. When full extension is reached, immediately lower the dumbbells slowly to the original position.

3. Repeat the movement, keeping in mind the stable position of the back against the bench.

Muscles Involved

Primary: pectoralis major, triceps, anterior deltoid

Secondary: biceps, rectus abdominis

⚠️**SAFETY TIP** For the physioball dumbbell press variation, the weight of the dumbbells should be reduced because of the relative instability of the physioball versus the bench, but after becoming comfortable with the movements, dumbbell weight can be added.

Running Focus

As mentioned earlier in the chapter, the muscles of the chest become fatigued by exercise in exactly the same way as do all other muscles, so developing these muscles through a simple exercise like the dumbbell press is both easy and beneficial. This exercise recruits the abdominal group more than the barbell bench press because the torso requires stabilization as a result of the independence of each dumbbell. It targets the pectoral muscle group and uses the abdominal group as stabilizers. The stronger the abdominal and pectoral group are, the better the posture of a distance runner in the latter stages of a race or training run, as well as the cardiovascular benefit of improved respiration. The better the upper-body posture of a runner, the more efficient the gait cycle is, aiding the runner by not wasting precious energy on poor running mechanics.

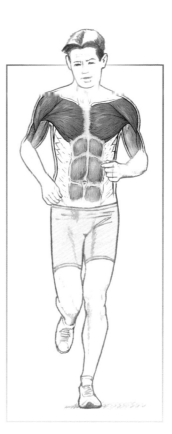

VARIATIONS

Rotated Dumbbell Press

This variation develops the sternal head of the pectoral group. It helps fully develop the pectoral group.

Dumbbell Press on Physioball

The use of the physioball enhances the role of the abdominal group as stabilizers for the exercise.

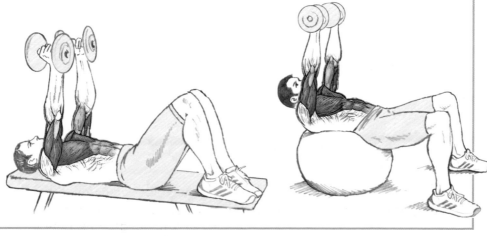

Incline Barbell Press

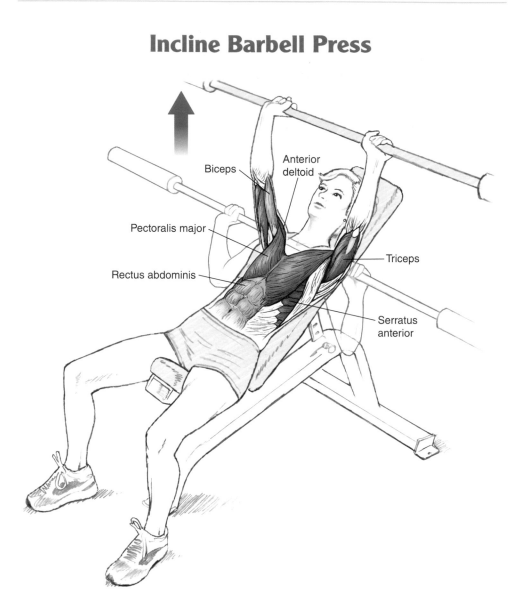

Execution

1. Lie on a 45-degree incline bench. With arms extended almost to their full extension, grip the barbell a little wider than shoulder width.
2. Fully extend the arms, removing the barbell from the rack. Lower the barbell in a straight line to the upper chest.
3. Press the barbell up, in a straight line, back to the original position without locking the elbows.

Muscles Involved

Primary: pectoralis major, triceps, anterior deltoid, serratus anterior

Secondary: biceps, rectus abdominis

⚠️ **SAFETY TIP** Use of a spotter is highly recommended to help with removing and placing the barbell back on the stays of the bench. Because of the inclined nature of this exercise, there is more shoulder involvement—specifically, the rotator cuff. If any pain is felt in the shoulder, discontinue the exercise and perform only the flat dumbbell press.

Running Focus

Similar to the dumbbell press in the muscles engaged, the incline press also involves the serratus anterior, adding to the development of the upper body. By adding variation to a strength-training routine through the use of different exercises that stimulate muscle growth in the same area, a runner can avoid becoming bored with a regimen. Because the strength-training component is meant to complement and enhance run training, performing new exercises helps keep the training fresh.

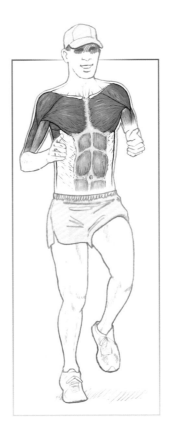

Dumbbell Fly

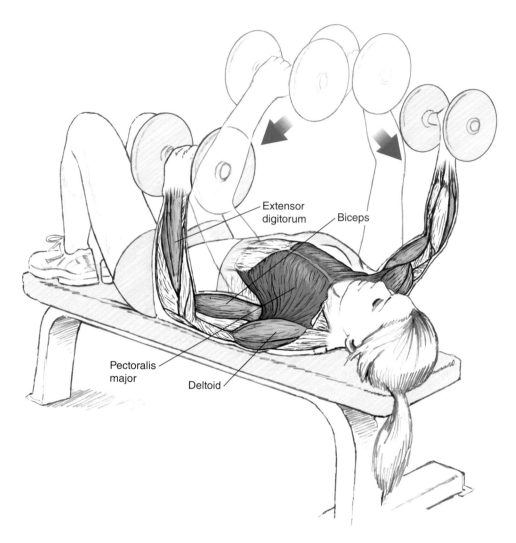

Extensor
digitorum

Biceps

Pectoralis
major

Deltoid

Execution

1. Begin by lying supine on a bench with legs steepled and feet on the bench. There should be a small, natural bend in the lower back so it does not touch the bench. Arms are extended perpendicular to the body with 5 to 10 degrees flex in the elbows. Hands grip the dumbbells, palms facing inward.

2. Lower the weight slowly, focusing on the stretch of the pectoral muscles while maintaining bent elbows, until the upper arms are outstretched and in the same plane as the bench top.

3. Return the weight to the starting position as if you were hugging a barrel. Control the dumbbells so they do not touch at the top, but are separated by 2 or 3 inches.

Muscles Involved

Primary: pectoralis major

Secondary: biceps, deltoid, extensor digitorum

⚠️**SAFETY TIP** Note that you begin the exercise with the dumbbells extended, not outstretched. Lifting the dumbbells to begin the exercise can be difficult if heavy weight is used, and starting in the outstretched position places the deltoids and biceps in an awkward position. Also, do not lower the arms past the plane of the bench top for fear of injury.

TECHNIQUE TIP
▸ When returning the weight to the overhead position, do not push the weight with your hands or overly engage your deltoids. Your pectorals should do the lifting.

Running Focus

The emphasis on strengthening the pectoral muscles has been noted in all the exercises listed in this chapter. However, the benefits of the dumbbell fly include the stretching of the pectoral muscles, specifically during the negative, or lowering, phase of the exercise. This stretching helps expand intercostal muscles between the ribs, allowing for better respiration. Essentially, the more the muscles of the chest are expanded, the easier it is to inhale oxygen. This is reflected in the large rib cages of elite marathoners like Ethiopian Haile Gebrselassie and American Ryan Hall. Their chests always seem expanded when they run, most likely to accommodate their exercise-enlarged lungs.

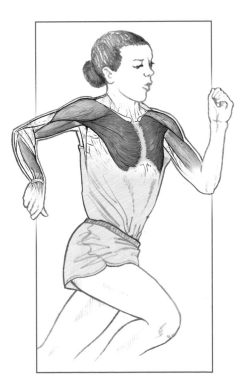

Push-Up

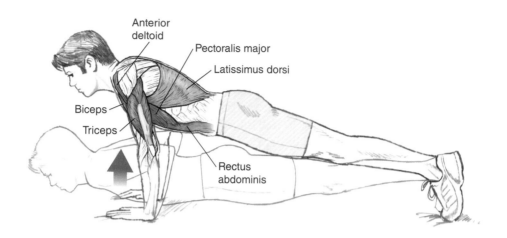

Anterior deltoid
Pectoralis major
Latissimus dorsi
Biceps
Triceps
Rectus abdominis

Execution

1. Start in a prone position, arms bent, slightly wider than shoulder-width apart, but in a straight line with the outsides of the shoulders.
2. Push away from the floor in a single, controlled movement, keeping your body in one slight upward plane (from feet to head) until your arms are fully extended. Exhale while performing the push-up.
3. Lower your body slowly by bending at the elbows until the chest is parallel and touching or near touching the floor. Inhale during this phase of the exercise.

Muscles Involved

Primary: pectoralis major, triceps, anterior deltoid

Secondary: biceps, latissimus dorsi, rectus abdominis

Running Focus

The push-up is the purest strength exercise. No machines. No weights (other than your own body weight). One fluid movement. It is not complicated unless you add variations (incline push-up and push-up on physioball), but it is a highly effective exercise for developing upper-body strength.

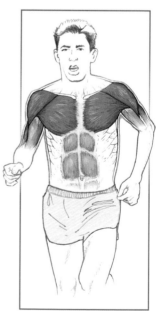

Push-ups benefit a runner by strengthening the upper body and abdominals, ensuring proper posture. The technique involved in completing a push-up is similar to the position of the upper body during running, so the exercise reinforces correct posture.

Multiple sets of push-ups can be done, but like any strength-training activity, push-ups should not be done daily, but following a rest period that allows for the mending of the muscle fibers used during the push-up session.

VARIATIONS

Incline Push-Up

Incline push-ups shift the emphasis of the exercise to the upper chest and the muscles of the shoulders. A greater number of push-ups can be performed, so incline push-ups are a good exercise to begin with if regular push-ups are difficult. Because the exercise is easier, you may be tempted to accelerate the motion, but resist this temptation. The rotator cuff is more involved in incline push-ups, and accelerating the motion could lead to a shoulder injury.

Push-Up on Physioball

Decline push-ups shift some of the emphasis to the upper back. Using a physioball while performing this exercise requires core stabilization, so this exercise aggressively targets secondary muscle groups. Try to keep your hips from sinking toward the ground during the execution of the push-up. Maintain a rigid posture. If this is difficult, use a smaller physioball, which makes the exercise easier.

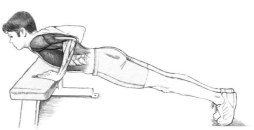

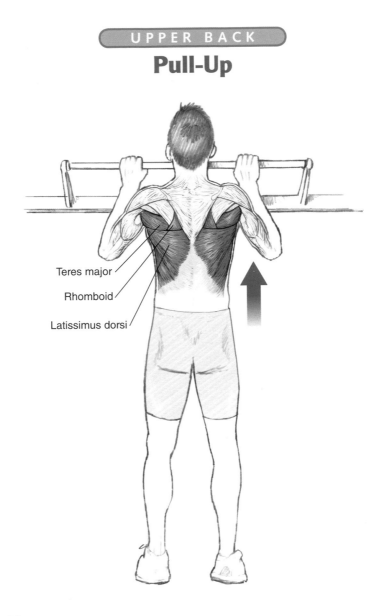

UPPER BACK
Pull-Up

Teres major

Rhomboid

Latissimus dorsi

Execution

1. Use an overhand (palms forward) grip and hang from the pull-up bar, getting a full stretch.
2. Pull your body weight upward using a fluid motion.
3. When the chin reaches bar height, lower your body in a controlled movement back to almost full extension of the arms. Feet should not touch the floor during repetitions.

Muscles Involved

Primary: latissimus dorsi, teres major, rhomboid

Secondary: biceps, pectoralis major

Running Focus

The pull-up is the yin to the push-up's yang. It is simply performed, but powerful in providing strength benefits. It helps strengthen the upper back, and as distance runners can attest, a strong upper back makes for better running posture during the later stages of a training run or long race.

The U.S. Marine Corps and other branches of the military use the pull-up (and push-up) to measure the fitness of their soldiers. A perfect score is 20 pull-ups in one minute.

Pull-ups are a difficult exercise. To aid in starting the exercise, stand on a box to begin the first rep. Do only the amount of pull-ups that can be done with a fluid, controlled movement. Do not wriggle or bounce.

Often pull-ups are called chin-ups. Some trainers distinguish between pull-ups and chin-ups based on the grip (palms outward or inward), but for others the difference is simply semantic.

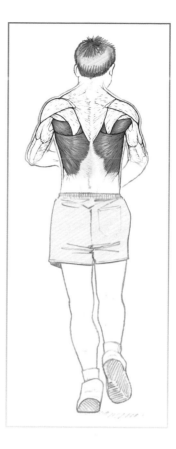

VARIATION

Reverse-Grip Pull-Up

Use an underhand (palms facing toward you), shoulder-width grip. Hang from the pull-up bar, getting a full stretch. Pull your body weight upward using a fluid motion. When the chin reaches bar height, lower your body in a controlled movement back to almost full extension of the arms. Feet should not touch the floor during repetitions.

The reverse-grip pull-up involves the biceps more than the overhand-grip pull-up. Given the relatively small size of the biceps, performing this exercise is more difficult than with the overhand grip because the biceps can fatigue quickly.

The two pull-up exercises can be alternated during a strenuous upper back workout, or they can be done on different days as part of a general workout.

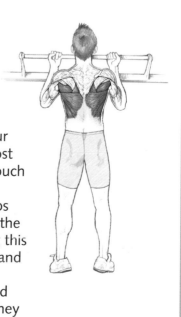

UPPER BACK

Machine Lat Pull-Down

Execution

1. Using a weight machine, face the bar with your legs under the pads and grip the bar using a wide grip. Arms are fully extended. Palms face away from the body. Your upper body is slightly rotated (shoulders back) to accommodate the exercise motion.

2. In one continuous motion, pull the bar down, with elbows back and chest out until the bar reaches the upper chest.

3. Gradually allow the arms to return to full extension while resisting the weight during the negative phase of the exercise.

Deltoid

Triceps

Teres major

Latissimus dorsi

Muscles Involved

Primary: latissimus dorsi, teres major

Secondary: triceps, deltoid

TECHNIQUE TIP

▶ The lat pull-down will cause significant muscle mass to develop in the upper back if heavy weight is used as resistance. It is recommended to perform the exercise with lighter weight than the maximum and to complete multiple sets of higher repetitions.

Running Focus

The lat pull-down motion is not a normal running movement, so how does this exercise aid running performance? Like the chest and upper back exercises previously illustrated, the lat pull-down helps performance by strengthening muscles (latissimus dorsi and teres major) that support and stabilize the body's thorax and aid in respiration and posture. The strengthening of the upper back helps counterbalance strength gained from performing the exercises targeting the chest, creating a torso that is balanced, and helps with maintaining an erect posture throughout a lengthy training or racing session. This is a good exercise to perform during the introductory phase of training.

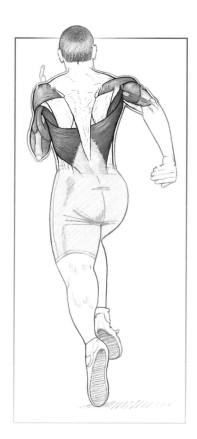

VARIATION

Reverse-Grip Lat Pull-Down

This exercise emphasizes the role of the biceps as well as the latissimus dorsi and teres major. We recommend completing this exercise on a day when strengthening the arms is the focus of the workout. If you perform the lat pull-down first, you may need to change the weight load to perform the reverse-grip variation since the latter minimizes the role of the larger shoulder and upper back muscles.

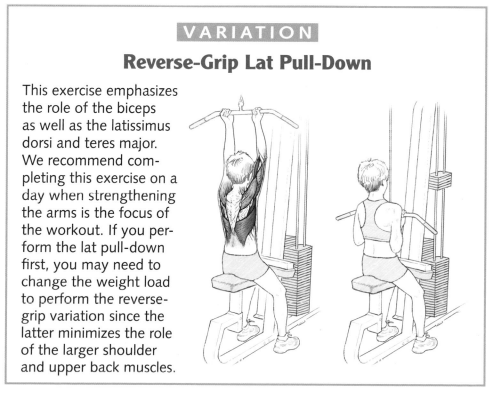

UPPER BACK

One-Arm Dumbbell Row

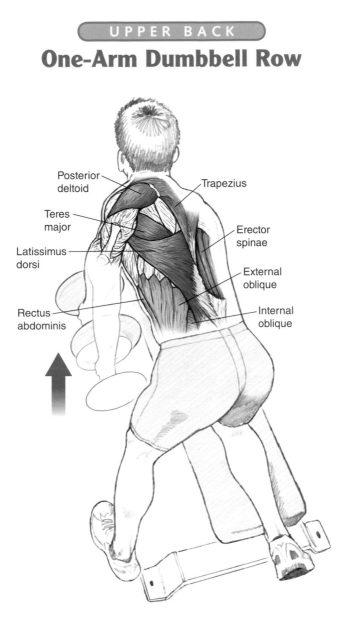

Posterior deltoid

Trapezius

Teres major

Erector spinae

Latissimus dorsi

External oblique

Rectus abdominis

Internal oblique

Execution

1. Kneel with one leg on a flat bench. Use the same-side hand (non-weight-holding hand) for support by placing it on the bench. The weight-holding hand is dropped below the bench top, arm extended down.

2. Grip the weight and, in a smooth, continuous motion initiated by the muscles of the upper back and shoulder, pull the dumbbell upward until the elbow is bent at a 90-degree angle. Exhale while performing the row.

3. Gradually lower the weight along the same path that the dumbbell traveled upward.

Muscles Involved

Primary: latissimus dorsi, teres major, posterior deltoid, biceps, trapezius

Secondary: erector spinae, rectus abdominis, external oblique, internal oblique

TECHNIQUE TIP

▸ **The movement of the exercise has been likened to that of sawing wood with a hand saw.**

Running Focus

This is an easy exercise to perform, and it benefits multiple muscles. Specifically, because a relatively heavy weight can be used (once good form is established), a lot of strength gains can occur. The development of the deltoid and trapezius will help with head position and arm carriage. Specifically, strength in these muscle groups will aid in developing a powerful arm carriage during track sessions, help fend off fatigue during longer workouts and races, and help maintain good running form during trail runs on difficult (rocky or hilly) terrain.

An important element of this exercise is the isolation of the upper back and shoulder muscles used. Although the abdominal group engages to stabilize the body, emphasis should be placed on the role of the latissimus dorsi, trapezius, deltoid, and biceps.

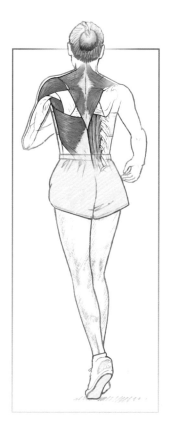

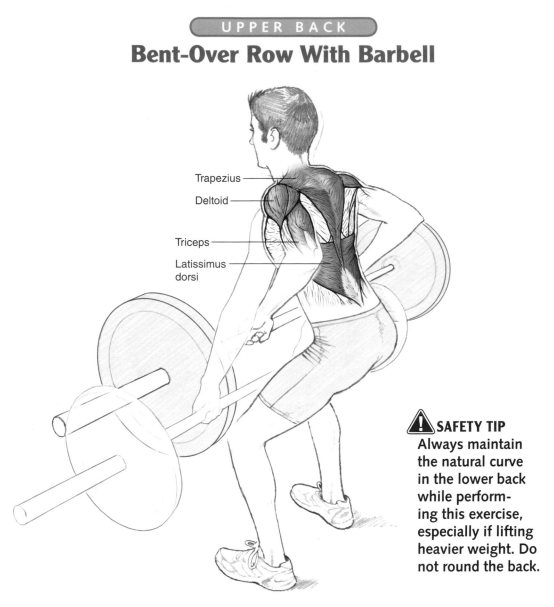

UPPER BACK

Bent-Over Row With Barbell

Trapezius

Deltoid

Triceps

Latissimus dorsi

⚠ SAFETY TIP
Always maintain the natural curve in the lower back while performing this exercise, especially if lifting heavier weight. Do not round the back.

Execution

1. Stand with legs shoulder-width apart, leaning forward at the waist, knees slightly bent, and arms hanging down, clasped to the barbell with a traditional grip, shoulder-width apart.
2. Pull the barbell to the chest, still in a bent position, until your elbows are bent parallel to the chest.
3. Return the weight to the starting position and repeat.

Muscles Involved

Primary: latissimus dorsi, trapezius

Secondary: triceps, deltoid

Running Focus

Muscle imbalances are prevalent in runners, predominantly between the four muscles of the quadriceps group, between the quadriceps group and hamstring muscles, and, more generally, between the legs (left versus right). Muscle imbalances of the upper body are often not addressed in strength training for runners because the practical shortcomings of such imbalances are not assumed to affect running perfor-mance. However, an imbalance between the "push" muscles of the chest and the "pull" muscles of the upper back can have a dra-matic impact on gait because the forward lean or lack thereof changes the degree of lift the quadriceps group can generate during the forward swing phase. A lack of lift as a result of too much forward lean can inhibit the speed of running, especially during faster-paced training.

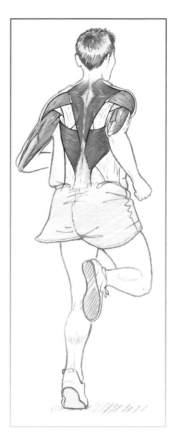

The speed not created by the normal lift of the gait cycle can be compensated for with faster turnover, but the resulting emphasis on aerobic capacity because of poor posture can have an adverse effect on performance if the athlete's aerobic fitness is subpar. Hence, the anatomy of running plays a major role in performance despite its seemingly second-ary role in fitness development. Specifically, if a large muscle group is strengthened (e.g., the pectorals through "push" exercises), the agonist muscles (in this case, those of the upper back) must be equally strengthened.

VARIATION

Wide-Grip Bent-Over Row With Barbell

A wider grip allows you to work the muscle at a different angle. In this case, it does not change the main muscle group worked. Some athletes with longer arms prefer the wider grip because it feels more natural. Maintain the natural curve in the lower back.

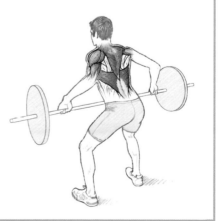

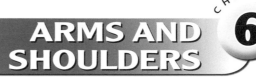

ARMS AND SHOULDERS

Sir Murray Halberg, a New Zealander, won the Olympic 5,000-meter run with a withered arm that was the result of an earlier sporting accident. Even people who lack arms are perfectly capable of running, and often do so very well. However, arms are a necessary part of a smooth running motion; each arm not only aids the balance of the runner, but also assists forward movement by acting as a counterbalance when the opposite leg drives away from the ground. To test this, try leading with your right hand and right leg at the same time—at best, it will feel unnatural; at worst, you will fall over! A further example is to watch a sprinter coming out of the blocks—a high knee lift accompanies exaggerated arm action for the first dozen strides, and then the arms continue to pump away for the rest of the sprint.

Distance runners would waste energy by driving the arms in this fashion; as economy of effort to save energy is all-important, so their arms hang fairly loosely, usually with elbows bent to 90 degrees or so with the hands relaxed beyond the wrist joints. Sprinters' fingers are straight and more tense as they drive each stride, a marked difference, so arms have a serious part to play in successful running, though in distinctly different manners for the type of run being attempted.

The arms are attached to the body at the shoulder joint, which is a shallow ball and socket to permit maximum movement through as close to 360 degrees as possible. This is quite effective, although the disadvantage of such mobility is an unstable joint that can be easily damaged. The ligaments that hold the shoulder in place have to be elastic enough to allow movement, so the stability of the joint relies on the strength of the retaining muscles.

It may be helpful to have a reminder of Newton's third law of motion: For every action, there is an equal and opposite reaction. If a muscle contracts and pulls the shoulder in one direction, then one or more other muscles will need to lengthen to allow this to happen. Strong muscles with good tone will tend to separate a joint if those opposing it are weak and undeveloped. This is never truer than with the shoulder joint.

The ball of the shoulder joint, at the upper end of the humerus, is located in the shallow glenoid labrum, or cavity, itself a part of the winged scapula that surrounds the posterior portion of the upper chest. From the runner's point of view, it is beneficial simply to know the muscles that maintain the position of the humeral head (figure 6.1) and which ones can

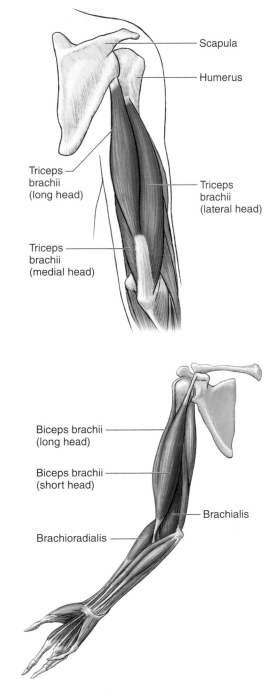

Figure 6.1   Upper arm: *(a)* back and *(b)* front.

be strengthened to improve running motion. The movement of the legs when they take large strides requires a similarly large movement of the arms backward and forward to balance the action. In sprinting especially, the arms and shoulders play a large part in propulsion, and a sprinter who is losing a race will often tense his or her shoulders as they go backward though the field. Anatomically, strong shoulders aid both strength and balance in the runner, so the exercises that follow are quite as important as those for the lower limbs. Tired arms and tense shoulders lead to a less fluent arm swing and a short stride that then uses unnecessary energy. The endurance that strength training of the upper limbs provides could make the hundredth of a second difference between success and a life-time of disappointment.

The outermost layer is formed by the triangular deltoid muscle. It arises from the clavicle, or collarbone, and part of the top of the scapula to cover the whole joint and be inserted into the middle of the humerus, where its contractions pull the arm out sideways into abduction. It opposes grav-ity. The complicated pattern of muscles underneath it have developed to enable movement in most planes. This matters little to runners, whose arms merely need to move no more than 45 degrees fore and aft, with minimal sideways movement. These muscles need to be strong rather than elastic. A complicated web holds the arm to the shoulder: The supraspi-natus braces the head of the humerus; the infraspinatus, subscapularis, and teres major and minor form a rotator cuff both to connect together and stabilize the shoulder.

Below the shoulder are the biceps, triceps, and brachialis muscles. Their primary function is moving the elbow joint, but some fibers are attached around the shoulder, giving even greater stability to that joint.

The extensor and flexor muscles of the forearm (figure 6.2) rotate the wrist inward and outward and also move the wrist and fingers. The flex-ors bend the joints in and the extensors open them out. More detailed knowledge of this anatomy is not the province of the runner, though their strength and flexibility undoubtedly are, so the exercises to promote this are all of relevance in increasing running speed.

Once again, any weakness will slow the runner, so the arms, particularly in power sprints, must have endurance equal to that of the legs. This explains why the physique of a sprinter's upper limbs is not unlike that of a boxer. Evolution has led to the use of arms when running, first to help stabilize the body and then to keep it upright as each leg moves. You should study a steeplechase runner in slow-motion replay to view how the arms help the body prepare for each takeoff, flight, and landing over the hurdles. Second, strong upper limbs not only aid in the production of full power when sprinting but also help the shoulders relax. When the shoulders tense, the runner inevitably slows. In short, a sprinter without arm movement is not a sprinter!

One other point to bear in mind is that the legs are unable to run with full efficiency if the arms are not involved in the running action. The effect

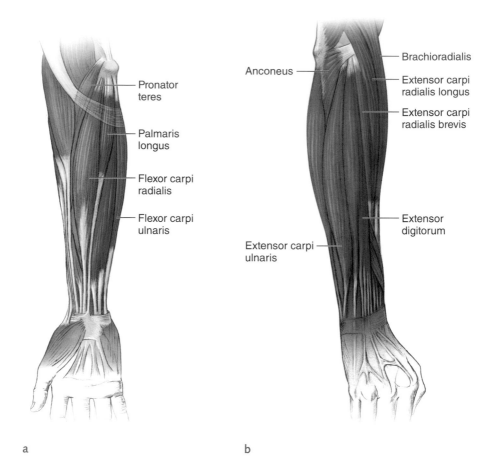

a   b

Figure 6.2   Forearm: *(a)* front and *(b)* back.

of this could be that strong legs want to speed up toward the end of a run, but are handicapped by upper limbs that have not been trained for the task. So when the arms fatigue, stride length and rate lessen and the runner slows.

Specific Training Guidelines

While performing biceps exercises, remember to keep your back straight; do not rock to help lift the weight. Choose a weight that does not hinder the smooth motion of the curl, and choose a lighter weight rather than a heavier weight to start. Also, keep your elbows fixed and close to your body, emphasizing the biceps and not the shoulders.

Most runners, if they do arm exercises at all, will emphasize the biceps exercises. We have emphasized the triceps to help balance the muscular strength of the arms. Both biceps and triceps exercises can be performed with smaller amounts of resistance. Since distance runners need to be able to swing their arms steadily in the later stages of a long run or race, not to suddenly produce power, the emphasis should be on a larger number of repetitions (18 to 24) because the emphasis is on muscular endurance. For mid-distance runners or sprinters, 8 to 12 repetitions of a heavier weight will suffice.

A good order for a sample arm workout would be the narrow-grip barbell curl, double-arm dumbbell kickback, and reverse wrist curl.

Alternating Standing Biceps Curl With Dumbbell

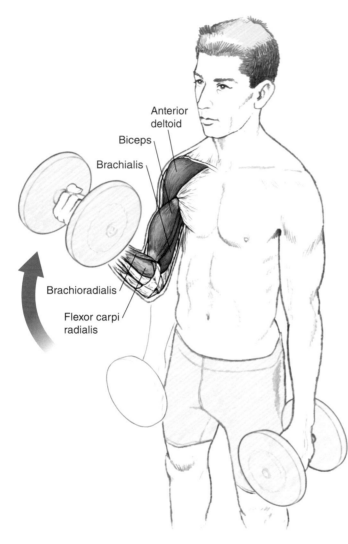

Anterior deltoid

Biceps

Brachialis

Brachioradialis

Flexor carpi radialis

Execution

1. Stand with feet shoulder-width apart and knees slightly bent. Arms should hang straight down from the shoulders, holding dumb-bells with the palms inward.

2. In one smooth motion, concen-trating on using the biceps and not the hand, curl one dumbbell upward, completing a full range of motion.

3. Using a slow, fluid movement, lower the dumbbell in the opposite direction of the curl. Feel the stretch as the dumb-bell returns to its starting position. Repeat the exercise with the other arm.

Muscles Involved

Primary: biceps, brachialis, anterior deltoid

Secondary: brachioradialis, flexor carpi radialis

TECHNIQUE TIPS

▶ **The upper arm should be fixed at the elbow; as the dumbbell passes 90 degrees, the upper arm should not move with it.**

▶ **Look sideways into a mirror, noting whether the elbow is staying fixed and there is little or no swaying (to aid in focusing on using the biceps brachii).**

⚠ **SAFETY TIP** This is a simple exercise that can go awry when too much weight is attempted. The ideal weight is heavy enough to provide resistance throughout each rep and set of reps, but not so heavy that poor form eventually occurs. Do not throw the weight by engaging your upper back muscles. The biceps dominates the movement.

Running Focus

It seems odd that runners need to develop biceps strength. Most distance runners appear emaciated, with thin arms and legs; however, this does not mean that their biceps are not strong. Developing strength is different from adding mass. The biceps exercise, when performed with enough resistance to stimulate strength gains and done with higher repetitions in conjunction with a strenuous running program, will promote functional strength endurance without added mass. Because the goal of the arms, for a distance runner, is to balance the runner from side to side and counterbalance the movements of the legs, the biceps should not fatigue during a grueling training or racing session. Strength endurance is paramount, and performing 12 to 18 repetitions and multiple sets of this exercise will help develop this type of strength.

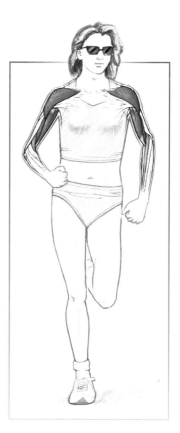

VARIATION

Barbell Curl With Variable-Width Grip

Barbell curls can be done with a normal shoulder-width grip, a narrow grip, or a wide grip. The narrow grip emphasizes the biceps brachii more than the other grips, while the wide grip incorporates the anterior deltoid (the large muscle encapsulating the shoulder). All three grips are appropriate, and a complete biceps workout can be completed by using just this exercise, incorporating one set of each grip.

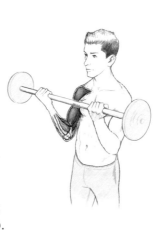

Alternating Standing Hammer Curl

Execution

1. Stand with feet shoulder-width apart. Arms hang straight down from the shoulders, holding dumbbells with the palms inward.

2. In one smooth motion, concentrating on using the biceps, not the hand, curl one dumbbell upward until it touches the shoulder, completing a full range of motion. The upper arm should be fixed at the elbow; as the dumbbell passes 90 degrees, the upper arm should not move with it.

3. Using a slow, fluid movement, lower the dumbbell in the opposite direction of the curl. Feel the stretch as the dumbbell returns to its starting position. Repeat the exercise with the other arm.

Biceps

Brachialis

Extensor carpi radialis brevis

Extensor carpi radialis longus

Muscles Involved

Primary: biceps, brachialis

Secondary: forearm extensors

⚠️ **SAFETY TIP** Avoid throwing the weight. Focus on the contraction of the biceps.

TECHNIQUE TIPS

▶ The upper arm should be fixed at the elbow; as the dumbbell passes 90 degrees, the upper arm should not move with it.

▶ Look sideways into a mirror, noting whether the elbow is staying fixed and there is little or no swaying (to aid in focusing on using the biceps brachii).

Running Focus

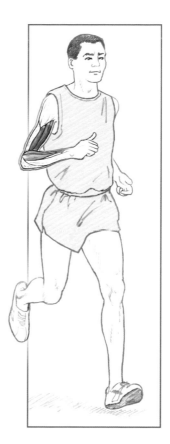

Similar in execution to the biceps curl—only the hand position is changed—the hammer curl develops strength in the biceps and, to a lesser extent, the brachialis. Performed during the same strength-training session at the end of the biceps set, the hammer curl is a fatigue-inducing exercise that also promotes joint flexibility because of its resistance over a full range of motion.

Often, runners complain of sore biceps during and after a race of a shorter duration with more intense effort. Because of the increased force of the arm carriage, a greater demand is placed on the muscles of the upper arm. By performing the biceps exercises, runners can stave off the fatigue during a race and shorten recovery time between reps during a workout.

VARIATION

Seated Double-Arm Hammer Curl

While seated on the edge of a flat bench, feet flat on the floor, back erect, and arms hanging down with a dumbbell in each hand, palms inward, perform the hammer-curl motion with both arms simultaneously. This exercise involves the coordination of both arms, and may cause fatigue a little quicker than when alternating arms.

Dumbbell Lying Triceps Extension

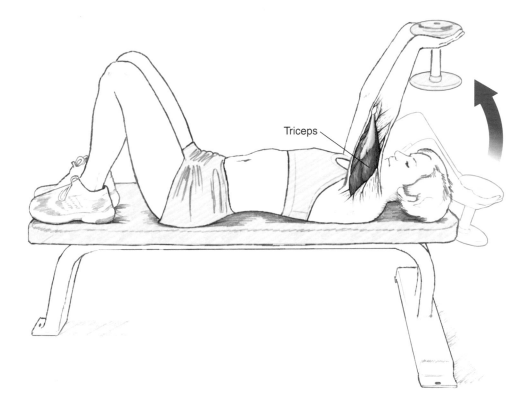

Triceps

Execution

1. Lie on a flat bench with both feet on the bench. The torso should be stable. Arms are bent 90 degrees at the elbow, shoulder-width apart. Hold a dumbbell of an appropriate weight with both hands, palms inward.
2. Extend the forearms to full extension.
3. Lower the arms to the initial position slowly, resisting the weight.

Muscles Involved

Primary: triceps

⚠️**SAFETY TIP** Have a spotter place the weight in your hands and hold the weight in place until you begin the exercise. If there is not a spotter, begin the exercise with the arms in the extended position, and perform the negative (lowering the weight) action as the first movement.

Running Focus

The introduction to this chapter emphasized the importance of the arms in balancing and counterbalancing during running. The triceps exercises listed in this section serve to balance the recommended biceps exercises, creating a well-developed and strengthened upper arm. The muscles of the forearm are involved as secondary movers. The only movement occurs at the elbow joint, precipitated by the engagement of the triceps.

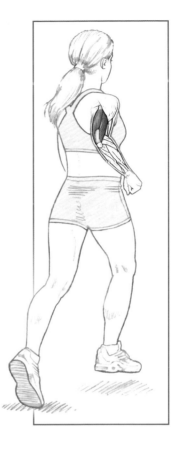

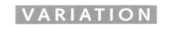

Barbell Lying Triceps Extension

Instead of using a dumbbell, using a barbell to perform the same exercise works well. Execute the exercise the same way, and follow the same safety instructions.

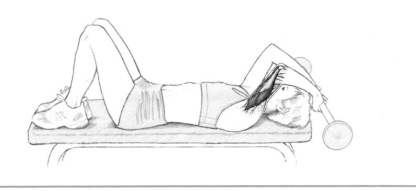

Single-Arm Dumbbell Kickback With Bench

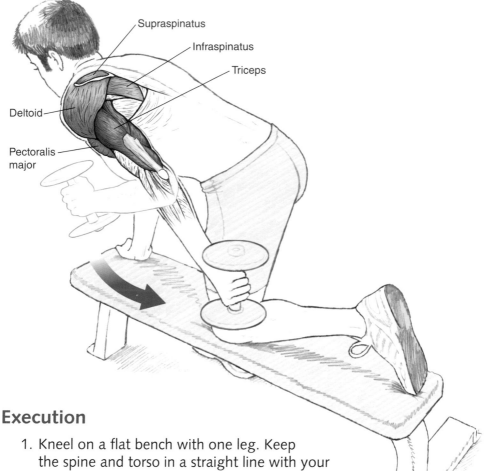

Supraspinatus

Infraspinatus

Triceps

Deltoid

Pectoralis major

Execution

1. Kneel on a flat bench with one leg. Keep the spine and torso in a straight line with your head. Establish a stable base of support with the non-weight-bearing hand pressed to the bench, and the opposite-side leg extended with the foot on the floor. The weight-bearing arm is bent at about a 90-degree angle with the palm inward.

2. Extend the forearm backward from the elbow, using the triceps muscles to instigate the movement in a slow, fluid fashion. Keep the elbow in a fixed position parallel to the torso, not higher. Exhale during this motion.

3. Upon straightening the arm, allow the weight to return the arm to 90 degrees by providing gentle resistance. Inhale during the return.

Muscles Involved

Primary: triceps

Secondary: infraspinatus, supraspinatus, deltoid, pectoralis major

TECHNIQUE TIP
▶ It is important not to vary elbow position during the exercise. Keep the elbow tight to the body and fixed. Try to avoid dropping the shoulder to help push the weight backward.

Running Focus

The dumbbell kickback is primarily a triceps exercise, but it recruits the infraspinatus and the supraspinatus muscles of the shoulder. Because the initiation of the arm swing during running takes place in the shoulder, strengthening the triceps and shoulder via this exercise helps ward off arm fatigue and bad posture, two energy-sapping scourges of good performance.

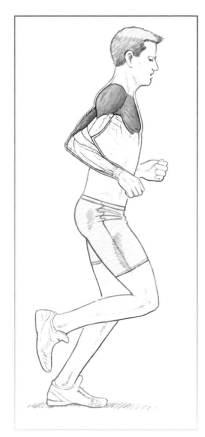

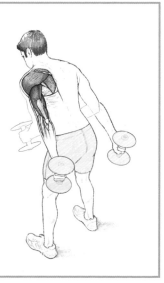

VARIATION

Double-Arm Dumbbell Kickback

The double-arm variation does not require a bench. From a standing position, bend over at the waist so your torso is close to parallel to the floor, feet shoulder-width apart, and grasp a dumbbell in each hand with the arms hanging downward. Perform the kickback movement with both arms simultaneously. The exercise uses the same muscles as the single-arm kickback using a bench, and will incorporate the core muscles of the abdomen and lower back to stabilize the body.

Machine Reverse Push-Down

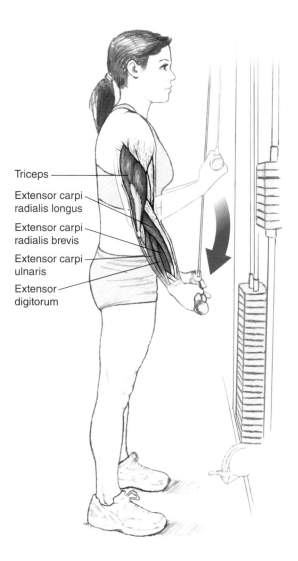

Triceps

Extensor carpi radialis longus

Extensor carpi radialis brevis

Extensor carpi ulnaris

Extensor digitorum

Execution

1. Standing with your feet narrower than shoulder-width apart, grasp the short, straight bar attached to a cable (on a pulley attached to the machine) with palms upward (underhand grip). The forearms are extended at approximately 75 degrees to the elbows, which remain fixed at your sides throughout the exercise.

2. In a smooth, uninterrupted motion, push the forearms downward in full extension, keeping the elbows fixed in their original position and close to the body. Exhale throughout the motion.

3. Allow the weight to return to the original position by resisting the pull of the cable gradually and in a smooth manner. Inhale during this part of the exercise.

Muscles Involved

Primary: triceps, forearm extensors

Running Focus

The reverse push-down mainly works the triceps, but it has the added benefit of also working the forearm muscles because of the underhand grip. This exercise marks a nice transition from the triceps-dominated extension and kickback into the next exercises, wrist curls, which predominantly work the forearm muscles. The triceps muscles and the extensor muscles of the forearms will fatigue quickly during the exercise as they do during a shorter distance race (5 to 10K), when using the arms becomes a means of propelling the legs during surges and effecting a finishing push.

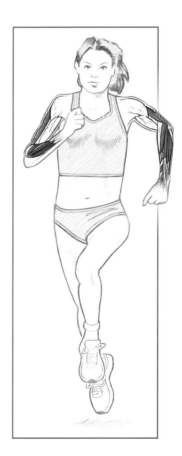

Wrist Curl and Reverse Wrist Curl

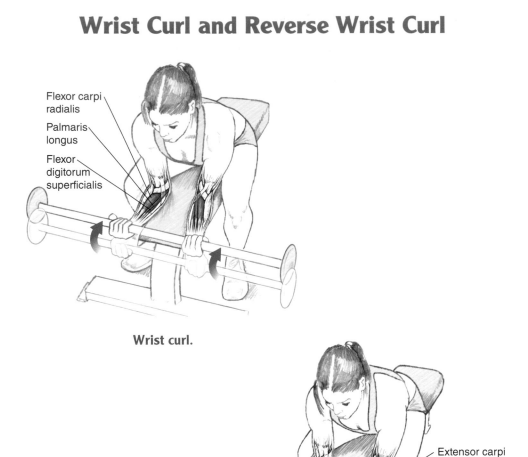

Flexor carpi radialis

Palmaris longus

Flexor digitorum superficialis

Wrist curl.

Extensor carpi radialis longus

Extensor digitorum

Reverse wrist curl.

Execution for Wrist Curl

1. Lean forward on a flat bench with your forearms resting on the bench. The wrists and hands should extend off the bench. Palms should be facing up with a barbell of a light weight resting forward of the palms with the fingers gently closed around the bar.
2. Raise the barbell by raising your hands, involving only the muscles of the forearms and hands, through a full extension.
3. Return the weight to its original position, gradually resisting the barbell as it moves downward.

Execution for Reverse Wrist Curl

1. Lean forward on a flat bench with your forearms resting on the bench. The wrists and hands should extend off the bench. Palms should face downward with a barbell of a light weight gripped securely by the palms and fingers.
2. Raise the barbell by raising your hands, involving only the muscles of the forearms and hands, through a full extension.
3. Return the weight to its original position, gradually resisting the barbell as it moves downward.

Muscles Involved

Primary: forearm flexors, forearm extensors

TECHNIQUE TIPS
▸ **Focus on a full stretch of the muscles, but do not allow the barbell to snap down.**
▸ **If it is difficult to rest your forearms on the bench, you can rest them on your legs.**

Running Focus

After gradually incorporating the extensor and flexor muscles into the strength-training routine, use wrist curls and reverse wrist curls to emphasize these muscles. During the course of a four-hour marathon, each arm will swing approximately 22,000 times. Although the movement is initiated by the larger muscles of the shoulders, the upper arms and the forearms are involved in the arm carriage. Specifically, each forearm is held at approximately 90 degrees to the upper arm to counterbalance the action of the opposite-side leg. During the course of 22,000 arm swings and four hours of being held aloft (fighting gravity), fatigue is bound to set in, creating a chain reaction of biomechanical adjustments resulting in poor form and wasted energy.

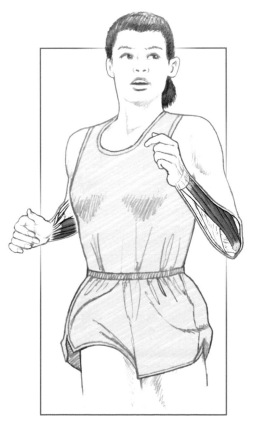

By performing the strength-training exercises for the arms, this fatigue and its chain reaction of bad results can be mitigated, if not eliminated—hence, less wasted energy, and hopefully faster times and better performances.

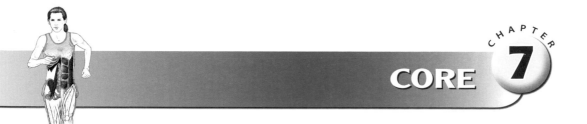

Running for pleasure was a long way down the list of priorities that determined how the pelvis would evolve in humans. The bones that form it are principally in place as a protective structure for the developing fetus, a need not shared by men, in whom a narrower pelvis forms the platform from which the legs unite with the rest of the body parts and have developed to accommodate locomotion.

Six major bones form the pelvis, two each of ilium, ischium, and pubis (figure 7.1a). Although these bones are solidly joined to each other with no discernable laxity, each ilium meets the lowest part of the spine, the sacrum, posteriorly at the large sacroiliac joints, where there can be considerable movement. This is most noticeable during childbirth, when hormonal influences cause the ligaments that bind the joint to relax to such an extent that the joint may become subluxed, or partially dislocated, with considerable instability and possible consequences for the female runner. Above the sacrum are the five lumbar vertebrae, which have an important function in keeping the whole skeletal structure stable. As well as these two joints, each pubis is linked at the front by the symphysis pubis at the lowest point of the abdomen. This is a more solid fibrous connection, but sometimes liable to damage in a slip or fall or as a result of chronic overtraining, for it forms the pivot and point of maximum force and corresponding weakness between the legs and torso.

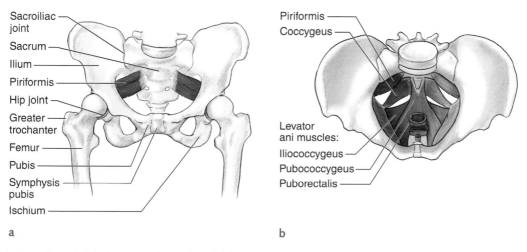

Sacroiliac joint
Sacrum
Ilium
Piriformis
Hip joint
Greater trochanter
Femur
Pubis
Symphysis pubis
Ischium

Piriformis
Coccygeus
Levator ani muscles:
Iliococcygeus
Pubococcygeus
Puborectalis

a

b

Figure 7.1 Pelvic bones and muscles: (a) bony structures; (b) pelvic floor muscles.

On the side of each ilium is a depression that forms the hip, known as a ball-and-socket joint. Its shape has developed in order to combine maximum stability with the greatest possible range of movement. The shoulder is similar but shallower and has a far greater likelihood of dislocation under load. The head of the femur forms the ball; movement of the joint is limited by the bony surrounds of the acetabulum, or socket, and also by the density and elasticity of the surrounding muscles and tendons.

If the pelvis is viewed from above as an oval-shaped clock, the two sacroiliac joints are fairly close together at the 11 and 1 o'clock areas, the hips at 4 and 8, and the symphysis at the 6 o'clock site. If one of these joints is moved, then another has to change position to compensate. This becomes important when running, for the pelvis is swung from side to side and twisted during the gait cycle, which has an effect on all the structures in and around it.

Forming a floor to the pelvis is the levator ani (figure 7.1*b*), which, for those with some knowledge of Latin, does just that. It lifts the anus and cradles all the other internal organs that fill the pelvis so that they do not collapse through the pelvic outlet. Weakness of the levator ani will predispose people to degrees of incontinence, and it is a muscle that requires training and toning just like any other. Running increases the pressure inside the abdomen, so any frailty may produce unwanted physical symptoms.

The other pelvic muscles have a dual function to stabilize and move the legs from their pivot at the hip joints. The stability is aided by some large ligaments, which are relatively inextensible, though with good breadth of movement. Running from the lumbar vertebrae and the interior of the ilium are the iliopsoas muscles, which pass through the pelvis, forming soft walls for the internal organs, to the inside of the femur below the hip joint. Over the lumbar vertebrae, they are counteracted by the erector spinae muscles, which stabilize the spine externally. The iliopsoas is a strong flexor of the hip and pulls the thigh up toward the abdomen.

The bulk of the buttock is formed by the glutei, three layers of muscle that slope down the outside of the back of the ilium at 45 degrees. Contraction of the outer layer, the gluteus maximus, extends and rotates the hip joint outward. It continues down the outside of the thigh as the tensor fasciae latae (see chapter 8 for more about this). The gluteus medius and minimus, underneath it, insert into the top of the femur at the greater trochanter, where their action is to pull the thigh outward, known as abduction, with the hip joint acting as a fulcrum.

Runners with low back pain are frequently diagnosed with piriformis syndrome. The piriformis muscle lies alongside the gluteus medius, and pain probably occurs because of its close proximity to and irritation of the sciatic nerve. It both stabilizes and abducts the hip joint.

Because the hip joint is so mobile, there have to be groups of muscles to counteract the forces produced by those that originate around and above the pelvis. These primarily pull the hip backward, abduct, and rotate it outward. The opposing muscles are those of the upper leg, which often have more than one function. The hamstrings— semimembranosus, semitendinosus, and biceps

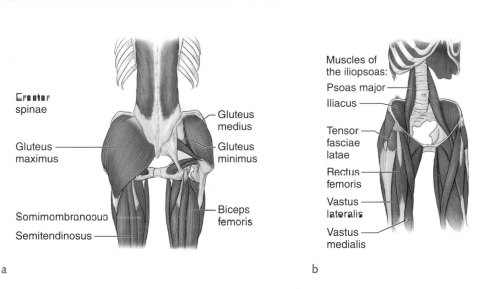

Figure 7.2   Lower core through upper leg: *(a)* back; *(b)* front.

femoris—all arise from the lower pubic bone (figure 7.2) and travel down the back of the thigh and behind the knee joint as its flexor (the lower limbs are discussed in more detail in chapter 8). Their upper leg function is to extend the hip backward. The opposite of abduction is adduction, and the three adductors, magnus, longus, and brevis, together with the gracilis, all pull the thighs together. They arise from the inside of the pubis and are inserted along the inner border of the length of the femur. As well as the iliopsoas, the rectus femoris and the other quadriceps muscles also extend over the hip joint, and when contracted, have a flexing action on the femur.

Muscles may be distinct entities, but often merge into one another and when dissected can be difficult to separate. The running action is repetitive, so that muscles with even slightly different functions may oppose each other during the running cycle and actually produce negative frictional forces. Where this may happen, a small fluid-filled sac called a bursa may form, the largest of which is over the greater trochanter, known as a trochanteric bursa. This may become inflamed and sore.

Returning to the pelvis and its adjacent organs, the abdomen, unlike the chest, does not have a bony architecture to stabilize it. The vertical height is maintained by the lumbar vertebrae. The responsibility for stability falls to the abdominal contents, which exert a counterpressure to a surrounding circular wall of muscles formed by the rectus abdominis, which extends from the base of the rib cage centrally down to the pubic symphysis and bone (figure 7.3). Outside this and lying diagonally are the external and internal oblique and the transversus abdominis muscles, which have three functions: to abduct and rotate the trunk, to flex the lumbar and lower thoracic vertebrae forward, and to contain the abdomen. When running, these muscles alternately lengthen and shorten as the pelvis moves not only from side to side, but also twists, rises, and falls relative to the surrounding body parts. In addition, they have

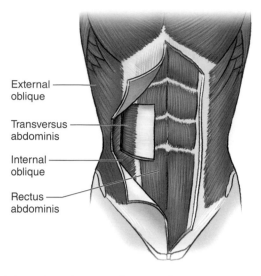

External oblique

Transversus abdominis

Internal oblique

Rectus abdominis

Figure 7.3   Rectus abdominis and surrounding muscles.

a function to aid respiration at high rates, working in conjunction with the diaphragm and ribs, which is particularly noticeable if the runner is reduced to panting. Thus, they have multiple roles, all of which may be required at the same time, and will perform better if well and thoroughly trained.

Rather than being active exercisers while running, the lower back muscles and lumbar vertebrae have more of a stabilizing passivity. First and foremost, they must maintain an upright posture, tempered by the need to accommodate for hills, where the upper body must lean backward or forward to counteract gravity upending the runner. The encircling musculature must allow rotation, body lean around corners, and lateral movement on any diagonally sloping surface, so they will contract and expand to maintain this stability. These complex movements have to coexist in conjunction with all the other variations in posture that occur as the legs move, the lungs breathe, and the abdominal contents shift to accommodate ingested fluid and nutrients during the run. Intrinsic strength, particularly of the muscles that surround the lumbar vertebrae, should be considered an essential in every runner because any weakness is liable to escalate into other areas.

Specific Training Guidelines

For the core exercises that require the movement of body weight only, multiple sets can be performed with many repetitions. All body-weight exercises should be slow and deliberate. Without extra resistance, the emphasis should be less on moving weight and more about perfect movement.

High repetitions are a great way for a runner to develop muscular endurance, which benefits long-distance runners; however, strength development to aid power only comes from using heavier resistance. Choosing what weights to use (when applicable) and how many or how few repetitions are to be performed is a function of the goal of the workout, and in the macro sense, the performance goal of the runner.

Core exercises should be performed at all stages of the training progression. Since many are body-weight bearing only, requiring no additional load, they can be performed three or four times per week.

LOWER BACK AND GLUTES
Back Extension Press-Up

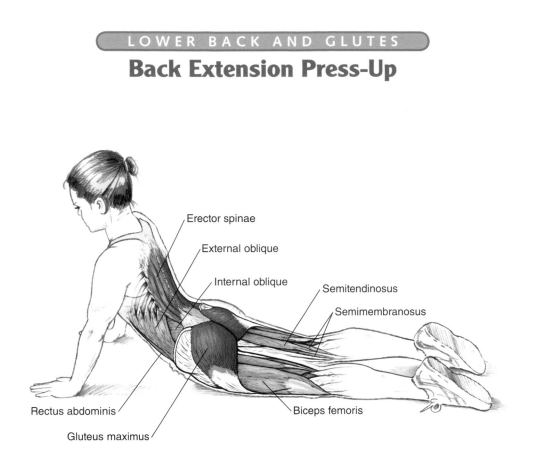

Erector spinae

External oblique

Internal oblique

Semitendinosus

Semimembranosus

Rectus abdominis

Gluteus maximus

Biceps femoris

Execution

1. Lie prone on the ground with arms in the push-up position and legs outstretched. Keep the body rigid and in a straight line.
2. Press up the arms only until the torso is off the ground. Hold this position for 10 to 15 seconds, breathing throughout.
3. Lower the arms, bending at the elbows, and return to the original position.

Muscles Involved

Primary: erector spinae, gluteus maximus

Secondary: hamstrings, rectus abdominis, external oblique, internal oblique

Running Focus

This a very simple exercise to perform. Not to be confused with a synonym for the push-up, the press-up extension of the lower back helps strengthen the muscles and tendons of the erector spinae, and acts as the antagonist for the rectus abdominis muscle. This exercise both strengthens and stretches the support structure of the sacral and lumbar spine, helping the pelvis rotate and twist properly, and mitigating the forward tilt of the pelvis if too many abdominal strengthening exercises have been performed, leading to an imbalance between the abdominals and muscles of the lower back.

Unfortunately, an emphasis on the core exercises can become an emphasis on the abdominals, with little attention paid to the muscles of the lower back and the glutes. Without strong glutes and a supportive lower back, the hamstrings often can't generate sufficient muscular power despite their having been strengthened properly. Essentially, the strongest muscles are only as strong as the weakest link on the kinetic chain allows.

The proper movement of the pelvis is critical in the gait cycle. A misalignment of the pelvis due to muscle imbalances between the abdominal muscles and the muscles of the lower back can cause injuries that impede running performance despite good cardiothoracic fitness.

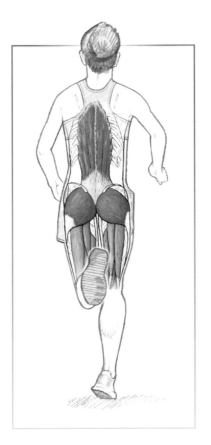

LOWER BACK AND GLUTES

Lumbar Hyperextension/ Alternating Arm and Leg Raise

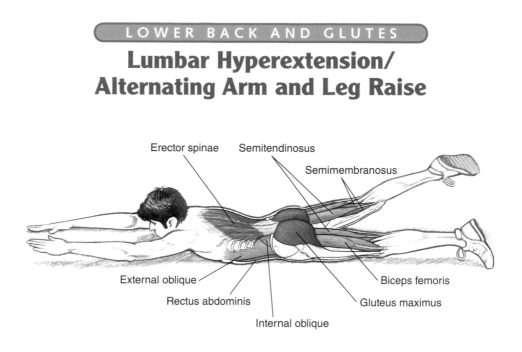

Erector spinae   Semitendinosus

Semimembranosus

External oblique

Rectus abdominis

Internal oblique

Biceps femoris

Gluteus maximus

Execution

1. Lie prone on the ground with arms and legs outstretched. Keep the body rigid and in a straight line.

2. Raise the left arm and the right leg three to four inches off the ground. Hold this position for 10 to 15 seconds, breathing throughout.

3. Lower the left arm and right leg, and raise the right arm and left leg simultaneously.

Muscles Involved

Primary: erector spinae, gluteus maximus

Secondary: hamstrings, rectus abdominis, external oblique, internal oblique

TECHNIQUE TIPS

▶ This exercise can also be performed on a Roman chair, where gravity plays a greater resistance role. Because Roman chairs are rarely around when you need them, performing this exercise on the ground works as well.

▶ All the movement should be generated by the muscles of the lower back and glutes.

⚠ **SAFETY TIP** Performing this exercise requires hyperextension of the back. Normally, this is not a problem, but for runners with chronic back pain or disc issues, press-ups are safer.

Running Focus

Lumbar hyperextensions can be performed in many ways. The goal of the lumbar extension is to strengthen and stretch the muscles of the lower back, glutes, and, to a lesser extent, the abdominals to help provide the appropriate pelvic tilt during the running gait cycle. A misaligned pelvis causes a chain reaction of misalignment, resulting in poor running form and wasted energy. Not only do the muscles of the back, abdominals, and glutes have to work in unison, but they also must work to balance each other and still generate enough strength to perform the exercise. This is very similar to how the core

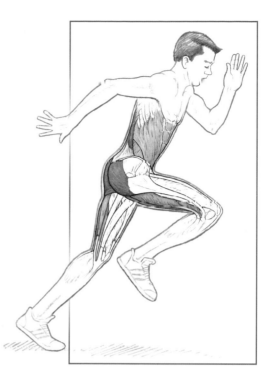

works when running. Because the pelvis is rotating and twisting, the core must dynamically stabilize, reacting to terrain shifts, turns, and missteps.

VARIATION

Lumbar Hyperextension on Physioball

Using a physioball changes the dynamic of the lumbar hyperextension. By only using one hand for balance (and, after mastery, no hands), there is a neuromuscular (proprioceptive) component added to the exercise. Ultimately, the goal of this exercise is to not include a balance hand. Balance can be maintained on the physioball from mastering the form of the exercise and strengthening the muscles of the core so that they can be activated when needed. Runners tend to overlook proprioceptive exercises because there is not much visible effort, rather small, subtle movements that help create more fluid running.

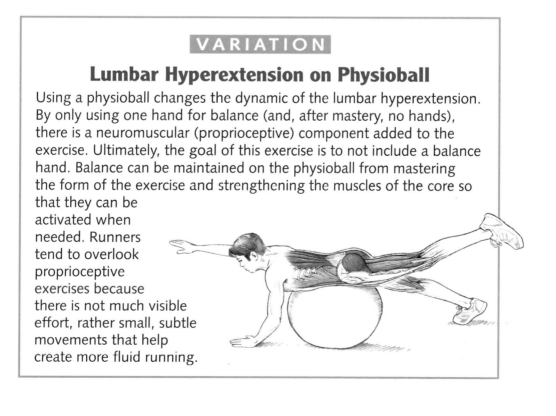

LOWER BACK AND GLUTES
Hip Abductor Machine

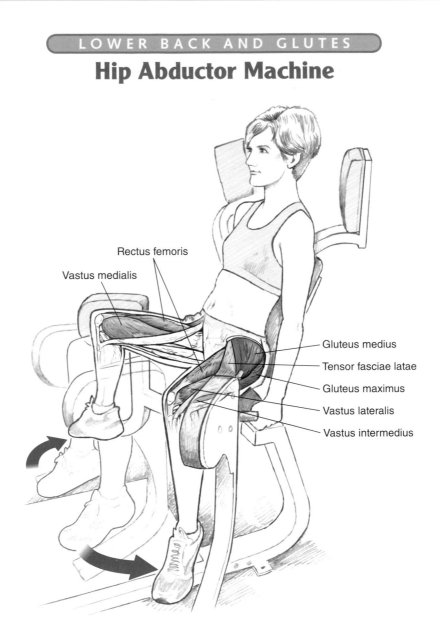

Rectus femoris

Vastus medialis

Gluteus medius

Tensor fasciae latae

Gluteus maximus

Vastus lateralis

Vastus intermedius

Execution

1. Sit in a proper seat position, with machine pads on the outsides of the knees.
2. Press outward using the abductor muscles (outsides of the legs). Emphasize reaching a full range of motion.
3. Return to the original position by gradually resisting the weight.

Muscles Involved

Primary: gluteus medius, gluteus maximus

Secondary: tensor fasciae latae, quadriceps

TECHNIQUE TIPS

▸ **The motion should be fluid, but with consistent effort throughout.**

▸ **The more upright the backrest, the more the emphasis on the gluteus medius.**

▸ **Avoid trying to overextend the exercise. Don't force the legs higher laterally than your hip naturally allows. Focus on pressing the legs apart using only the targeted muscles of the gluteus.**

Running Focus

The abductor exercise can be done during the same workout as the adductor exercise; it is easy to change the pad positions on the machine, but its emphasis on the glutes makes it a better fit with the exercises for the glutes and lower back. Many runners, especially those who underpronate, complain of piriformis pain at some point in their running careers. Because of its location, the piriformis muscle is difficult to stretch. However, abduction exercises aid in preventing and treating piriformis pain and sciatica by stretching and strengthening the gluteus medius, which is connected.

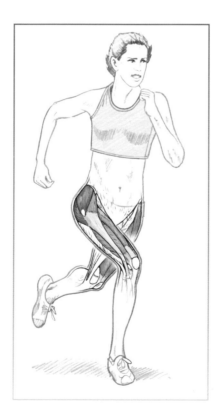

Floor Sit-Up

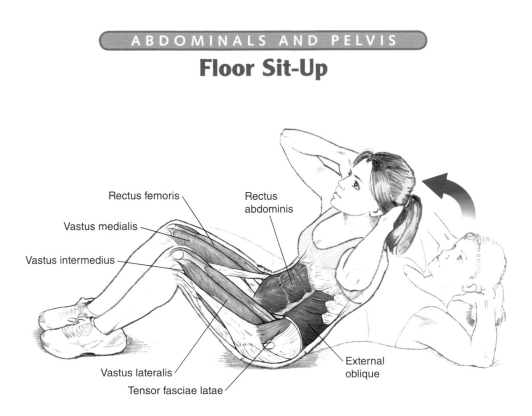

Rectus femoris

Vastus medialis

Vastus intermedius

Rectus abdominis

Vastus lateralis

Tensor fasciae latae

External oblique

Execution

1. Lie on the back with knees steepled, feet pressed to the floor, and hands gently touching the back of the head, but not clasped.

2. Raise the torso by rounding the back one vertebra at a time while pressing the pelvis down to floor. Raise the torso only 45 degrees before lowering the back to the floor.

3. Inhale, and gradually lower the torso to the floor one vertebra at a time.

Muscles Involved

Primary: rectus abdominis, external oblique

Secondary: quadriceps, tensor fasciae latae

TECHNIQUE TIP

▸ Sit-ups can be performed with a partner holding down the feet of the person performing the exercise. It makes the exercise easier, but allows more reps to be performed.

⚠ **SAFETY TIP** Don't clasp, but gently touch the hands behind the head because it is easy to pull the head and torso up by using the muscles of the arms.

Running Focus

Because the quadriceps and hamstrings counterbalance each other, so do the muscles of the abdominals and lower back. To avoid muscle imbalances and potential injury, it is important to perform abdominal exercises after performing the strength-training exercises for the lower back described in the first part of this chapter. The sit-up should not be performed for speed, but in a relatively quick, fluid manner. The lowering of the torso should be done slowly, with attention to the work the abdominals are doing.

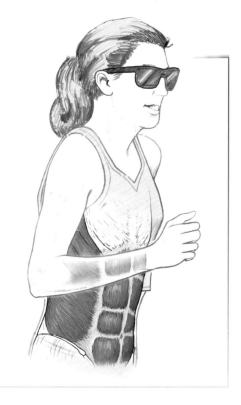

The rectus abdominis is the dominant muscle affected by sit-ups. It controls the flexion of the abdomen. Because almost all abdominal exercises work the rectus abdominis, a single set to failure can make up the start of an abdominal set.

The proper movement of the pelvis is critical to the gait cycle. A misalignment of the pelvis due to muscle imbalances between the abdominal muscles and the muscles of the lower back can cause injuries that impede running performance despite good cardiothoracic fitness.

VARIATION

Oblique Twist

A simple variation on the sit-up involves twisting the torso using the oblique muscles by attempting to touch the elbow to the opposite hip. A set of 12 can be done all on one side and then the other, or each rep can alternate sides.

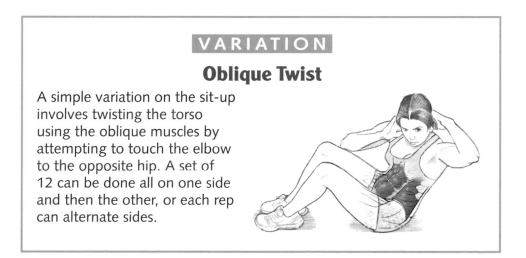

ABDOMINALS AND PELVIS

Hanging Leg Raise

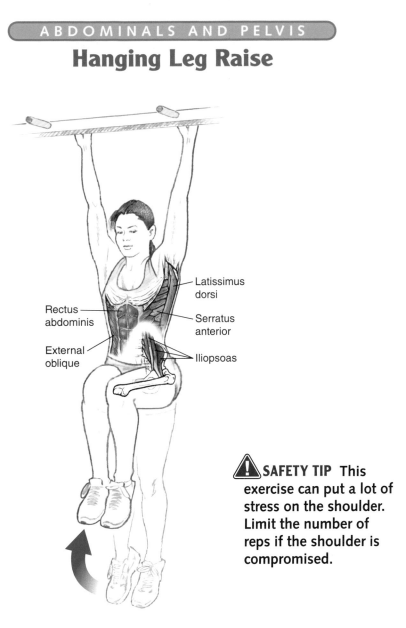

Latissimus dorsi

Rectus abdominis

Serratus anterior

External oblique

Iliopsoas

SAFETY TIP This exercise can put a lot of stress on the shoulder. Limit the number of reps if the shoulder is compromised.

Execution

1. Hang from a pull-up bar with palms facing forward. Emphasize lengthening, feeling gravity exerting its force on your spine.
2. Using a controlled movement, bring the knees up toward the chest. Keep the torso from swinging.
3. Gradually return to full extension and continue to repeat.

Muscles Involved

Primary: rectus abdominis, external oblique, iliopsoas

Secondary: latissimus dorsi, serratus anterior

Running Focus

The hip flexor muscles, specifically the iliopsoas, fatigue greatly during the course of a long run or race on a course that has the same terrain throughout. The repetitive nature of running is exacerbated with few terrain changes, and smaller muscles fatigue quickly. By strengthening the iliopsoas and the other hip flexors, runners can delay the onset of this fatigue. Also, when the terrain is hilly, requiring a lot of lifting throughout a run, weaker muscles will fatigue quicker, and gaining solid footing becomes harder.

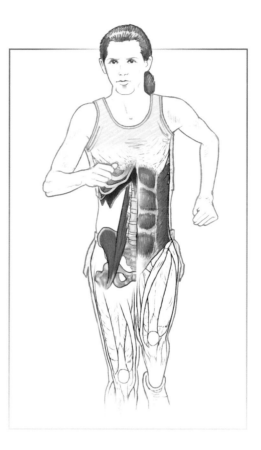

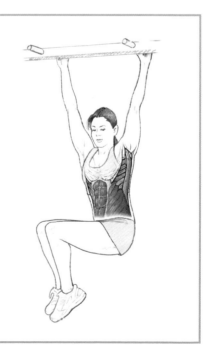

VARIATION

Hanging Leg Raise With Twist

The standard hanging leg raise affects the external and internal oblique, but adding a twist to the side increases the role of these abdominal muscles that are responsible for rotation and lateral flexion of the torso. As was mentioned in the introduction to this chapter, the oblique muscles help to twist, allowing for terrain adjustments, and they aid respiration by working in conjunction with the diaphragm and ribs.

Dumbbell Side Bend

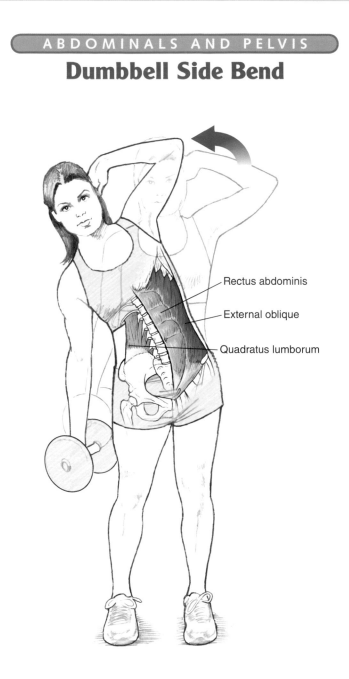

Rectus abdominis

External oblique

Quadratus lumborum

Execution

1. Stand with good posture, feet shoulder-width apart. Hold a dumbbell in one hand with the arm extended downward. The other hand is placed behind the head with the elbow out.

2. Bend at the waist in the direction of the hand holding the dumbbell, allowing the weight to pull the side down gradually.

3. Complete a set of 12 reps and then switch the dumbbell to the other hand and repeat.

Muscles Involved

Primary: external oblique

Secondary: rectus abdominis, quadratus lumborum

Running Focus

Balancing the abdominal muscles is the goal of this exercise. Most abdominal exercises focus on the large muscle of the abdominals, the rectus abdominis. The side-to-side movement of this exercise helps develop the external oblique, also strengthened in the hanging leg raise with twist. The strengthening of the external oblique helps minimize the side-to-side listing at the end of a fast race or hard effort in a speed workout. Because the smaller muscles of a large muscle group—that is, the abdominals—fatigue easier than the large rectus abdominis, it is important to do exercises that specifically target the smaller muscles so that they maintain their relative strength and do not become dominated by the larger muscle.

The practical application of this exercise is to eliminate the side-to-side rocking of the upper body during the gait cycle. While a leg length discrepancy could cause this rocking, the usual culprit is poor abdominal strength, especially weak oblique muscles. The inability of the abdominal muscles to maintain erect posture causes an awkward side-to-side motion generated by a pelvis that is not aligned.

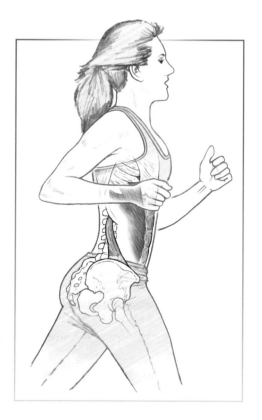

ABDOMINALS AND PELVIS
Single-Leg V-Up

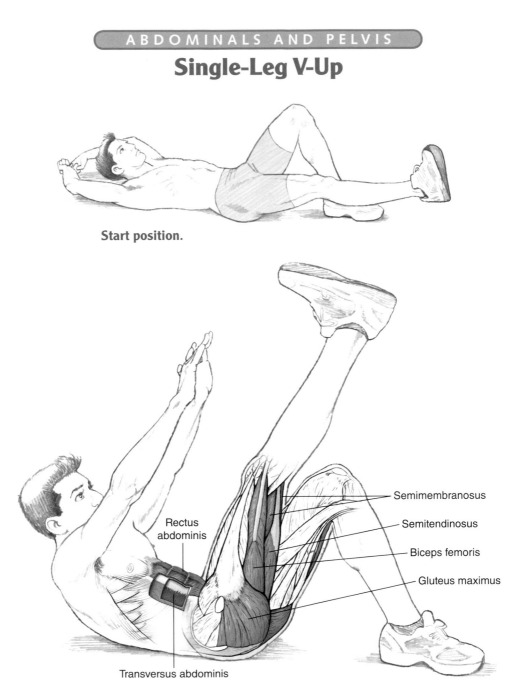

Start position.

Execution

1. Lie flat on the back with your hands reaching back behind your head. One leg is steepled and the other is raised approximately six inches off of the ground.

2. Leading with the chin and chest, engage the abdominals, raising up as in a sit-up, but also raise the leg that is off the ground, meeting the hand at its apex.

3. Recline to the initial position.

Muscles Involved

Primary: rectus abdominis, transversus abdominis, iliopsoas

Secondary: hamstrings, gluteus maximus

Running Focus

This exercise is dynamic and quickly fatigues the abdominal muscles and the iliopsoas. Because of the incorporation of both the upper body and lower body, there is more of a whole-body movement that more closely resembles a running movement than some of the other exercises in this chapter. Performed to failure, this exercise and its variation with a medicine ball can be an entire abdominal workout, especially if done as the final exercise in a strength-training session.

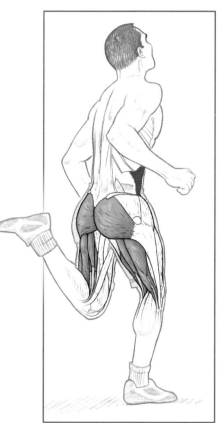

VARIATION

Single-Leg V-Up With Medicine Ball

The use of the medicine ball works the abdominals harder because of the added weight. Since the medicine ball is held away from the abdominals, even a five-pound ball feels heavy as a result of its distance from the fulcrum (the abdominal muscles). Also, the coordination of the movement with the added weight helps develop coordination, a skill not gained when just running in a forward motion.

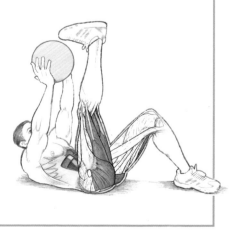

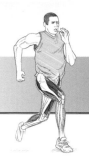
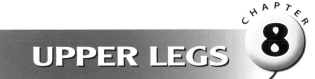
There is no real division between the core and the upper leg; all the limbs merge seamlessly into each other. Some of the pelvic muscles help movement and stability of the leg, and vice versa. The same occurs at the knee, where muscles are described as crossing over two joints, so they influence the action and steadiness of the joints. The upper leg (figure 8.1), or femur, is inserted via the hip joint into the pubis and ischium. The other bone of the upper leg, the patella (knee joint), is really a pulley. It runs in a groove at the lower end of the femur to help guide the extending forces of the quadriceps muscles around the knee.

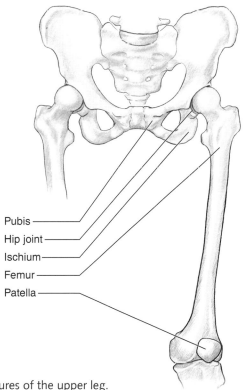

Pubis
Hip joint
Ischium
Femur
Patella

Figure 8.1 Bony structures of the upper leg.

The primary function of the quadriceps group (figure 8.2*a*) is to extend the knee. From the outside to the center line, the vastus lateralis, rectus femoris, vastus intermedius, and vastus medialis combine at the superior pole of the patella and straighten the knee joint with a pull through the patellar tendon on the upper part of the tibia. Contraction of this, the largest muscle group in the body, also pulls the knee toward the chest. It is particularly relevant to the sprinter, who gains extra stride length with big quadriceps contractions; however, this high knee lift wastes energy in a long-distance run, so the hip and knee have much smaller ranges of motion when covering longer distances. The role of the quadriceps in the running action is therefore twofold, though the intent of both movements is to increase the stride length (see figure 3.2 on page 23). If at the same time the knee is fully extended and the quadriceps muscles exert the maximum flexion to the hip, not only is the stride length maximized, but the added time in the air will also allow the momentum already generated to propel the body farther forward.

Much the same goes for the hamstring muscles (figure 8.2*b*), which also span the two joints but act in an opposite manner to both extend the hip and flex the knee. The semimembranosus, semitendinosus, and biceps femoris have some congruity in the center of their bulk, having arisen from different points within the pelvis, but then separate behind the knee and are inserted into the rear of the tibia and fibula. Contraction of the hamstrings drives both the upper and lower leg backward, a movement that tends to be exaggerated in a sprinter (see figures 3.3 and 3.4 on pages 24 and 25). Increased knee flexion would be inefficient to a distance runner; a greater percentage of the hamstring motion for a distance runner occurs at the hip.

It may be helpful to consider each full hamstrings group as two separate half muscles. This may sound paradoxical, but although it is the upper portion that links over the hip joint as an extensor muscle, the lower portion both flexes and limits extension of the knee. There is, of course, no actual physical distinction within the muscle groups when they are microscopically examined; the difference is purely functional. In the distance runner the hamstrings have a limited range of motion over both the hip and knee joint, although their contraction is very powerful over these small angles.

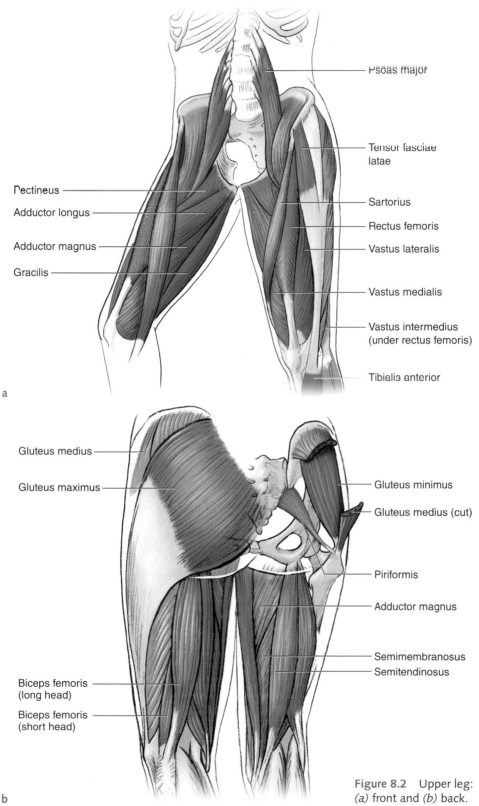

Psoas major

Tensor fasciae latae

Pectineus

Adductor longus

Adductor magnus

Gracilis

Sartorius

Rectus femoris

Vastus lateralis

Vastus medialis

Vastus intermedius (under rectus femoris)

Tibialis anterior

a

Gluteus medius

Gluteus maximus

Gluteus minimus

Gluteus medius (cut)

Piriformis

Adductor magnus

Semimembranosus
Semitendinosus

Biceps femoris (long head)

Biceps femoris (short head)

b

Figure 8.2 Upper leg: (a) front and (b) back.

It may seem strange that the knee needs to be able to twist, but how else would a runner turn corners or cope with uneven terrain? The knee (figure 8.3) has two collateral ligaments on the inside and outside that allow it to hinge to and fro, but rotation depends on the half-moon-shaped menisci, also known as cartilages, which are placed between femur and tibia and spread weight through the knee joint. They also allow the bones to twist on each other. An anterior and posterior cruciate ligament within each knee, placed in a crosslike shape, obstruct excessive forward and backward movement of femur and tibia on each other. It should be stressed, however, that these ligaments are there to guide knee movement and play only a small part in maintenance of knee stability, which depends mostly on the strength of the muscles.

The thigh muscles need both strength and flexibility, each of which can be improved by exercise. The maintenance of a balance between the two is also vitally important because being muscle-bound will do little for pliability; the converse is equally true in that lack of muscle bulk will cause relative weakness.

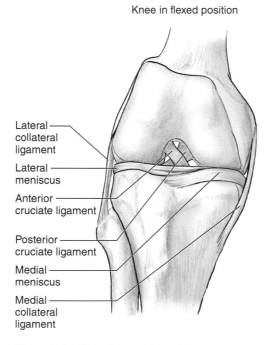

Figure 8.3   Knee ligaments and tissue.

Specific Training Guidelines

Protection of the knee joint while performing some of the following upper leg exercises is an important consideration. Because both the quadriceps and hamstrings groups of muscles attach to the knee, and the knee joint twists to adapt to terrain variations, turns, uphills, and downhills, there is constant stabilization and relaxation of the joint. The lunge exercises are difficult to perform initially, so care must be taken to perfect the motion with lighter weight before increasing the resistance. A machine-aided exercise helps protect the joint, but it has a fixed range of motion that does not make it the best functional exercise.

The exercises listed for the upper legs are good introductory and strength (threshold) phase exercises. However, they should not be done during the final phase of training, which emphasizes $\dot{V}O_2$max. During the final phase, substitute the plyometric exercises listed in chapter 12 to meet a runner's needs without overly fatiguing the muscles.

Hip Adductor Machine

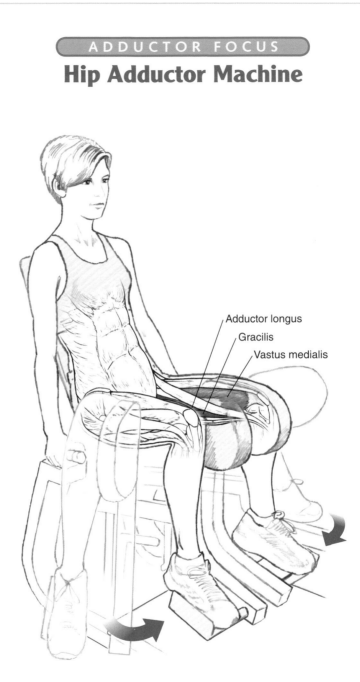

Adductor longus

Gracilis

Vastus medialis

Execution

1. Sit in a proper seat position, with machine pads on the insides of the knees.
2. Squeeze inward on the pads. The motion should be fluid but with consistent effort throughout.
3. Return to the original position by gradually resisting the weight.

Muscles Involved

Primary: adductor longus, adductor brevis, adductor magnus, gracilis
Secondary: vastus medialis

TECHNIQUE TIP

▸ **Avoid pushing the weight with the feet. Focus on bringing the
legs together with the adductor muscles.**

Running Focus

The adductor exercise can be used in
a strength-development regimen or as
a rehabilitative regimen that requires
ancillary muscles to be developed without undue stress on the knee joints.
Many knee problems are caused by
an imbalance of the four quadriceps
muscles, which cause tracking issues
for the patella. The adductor exercise
strengthens the adductor muscle group
specifically and the vastus medialis
secondarily, preventing the patella
from tracking too laterally. Developing
strength in the adductor group and the
quadriceps muscles of the upper leg
aids in the powerful extension during
the propulsive phase of the running
gait. To prevent imbalances in the
quadriceps, perform the abductor exercise on the same piece of equipment,
as described in chapter 7.

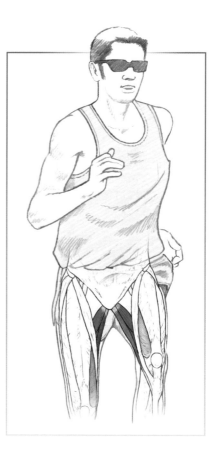

QUADRICEPS FOCUS
Machine Leg Extension

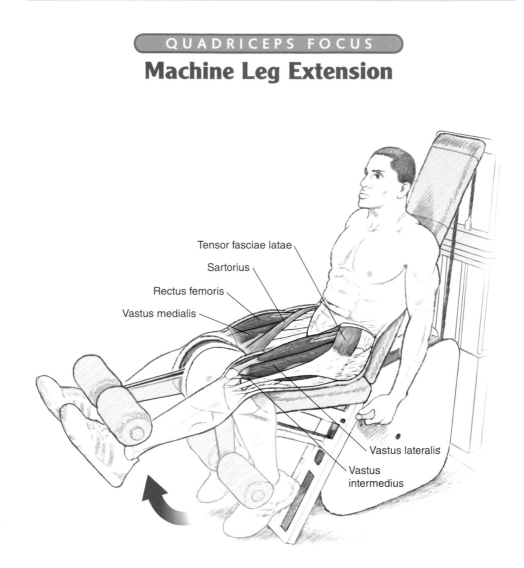

Tensor fasciae latae

Sartorius

Rectus femoris

Vastus medialis

Vastus lateralis

Vastus intermedius

Execution

1. Sit in the leg extension machine in the appropriate position. Keep the knees in line with the fulcrum of the weight lever and the back straight. Grasp the handles on both sides of the seat, but do not squeeze.

2. After choosing an appropriate weight, extend, but do not hyperextend, both legs through a full range of motion with a fluid motion.

3. At full extension, lower the legs gradually, resisting the weight while inhaling deeply.

Muscles Involved

Primary: quadriceps

Secondary: tensor fasciae latae, sartorius

TECHNIQUE TIP
> ▸ **Avoid hyperextending the knees and rocking the body to help lift the weight.**

Running Focus

The machine leg extension is a fantastic exercise because it is simple to perform and has a great impact on quadriceps strength. It develops the four muscles of the quadriceps equally (rectus femoris, vastus lateralis, vastus medialis, and vastus intermedius) and aids in keeping the patella tracking correctly. For runners suffering from a patellofemoral injury, the full extension needed for this exercise will unduly stress the patella. To help develop the quadriceps, a modified version of the exercise using a short arc (only the final 15 to 20 degrees of the exercise) helps off-load the patella. This exercise is a must during the introductory phase of training due to its general strength-building power.

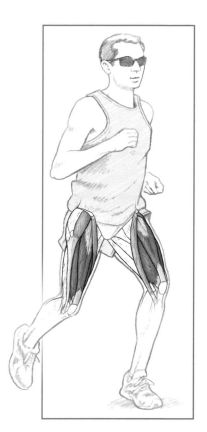

VARIATION

Machine Leg Extension With Short Arc

The leg extension with short arc variation is an excellent exercise for developing quadriceps strength if there is knee pain due to patellofemoral syndrome. The only drawback is that it is not a full range-of-motion exercise; however, once the knee pain dissipates, the full extension exercise can be completed.

HAMSTRING FOCUS

Machine Lying Hamstring Curl

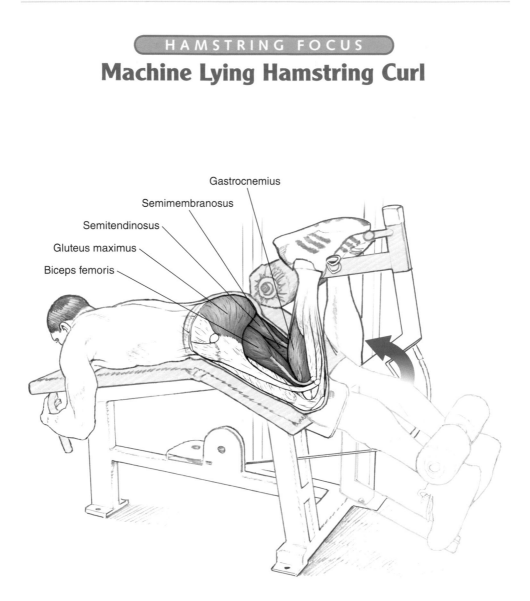

Gastrocnemius

Semimembranosus

Semitendinosus

Gluteus maximus

Biceps femoris

Execution

1. Lie prone on a hamstring curl machine. The pads of the machine are situated at the Achilles tendon. Hands are outstretched, holding onto the handles of the bench. Keep the head centered with the chin slightly off the bench.

2. Focusing on the hamstring muscles, slowly but fluidly pull the weight upward.

3. Return the weight to the starting position by gradually resisting the downward motion of the lever.

Muscles Involved

Primary: hamstrings

Secondary: gluteus maximus, gluteus minimus, gastrocnemius

⚠️ **SAFETY TIP** Some common mistakes made while performing this exercise are pulling strongly on the handles to help aid the motion of the exercise, lowering the weight too quickly, and slamming the weight into the glutes to finish the repetition.

Running Focus

As the counterpart to the machine leg extension, the lying hamstring curl works the large muscles of the hamstrings, helping to balance the quadriceps muscles of the front of the leg. The hamstrings come into play during the recovery phase of the gait cycle, as the lower leg bends at the knee, pulling the leg upward toward the glutes. The hamstrings group is not as strong as the quadriceps group, but it must be diligently strengthened or an imbalance between the quadriceps and hamstrings could occur. It is not common for distance runners to experience hamstring tears or pulls, but it is common for distance runners to suffer from hamstring tightness because of problems in the lower back. Also, many knee injuries are related to weak hamstrings.

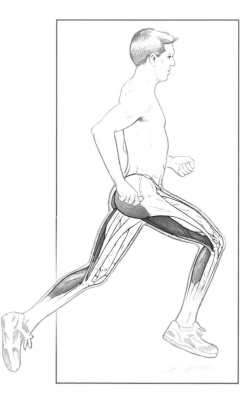

One complaint about the hamstring curl is that it works only the hamstrings and not the hamstrings and glutes, which work together in the gait cycle. While true, this is less significant if the exercise is performed in the base, or introductory, phase of training, where the emphasis is more on general strengthening and less on functional work, and where other exercises can work the glutes.

Dumbbell Lunge

TECHNIQUE TIP
▸ Do not attempt too much weight when first performing the exercise. Balance and flexibility play a large role in performing the movement, so practice good technique before adding weight.

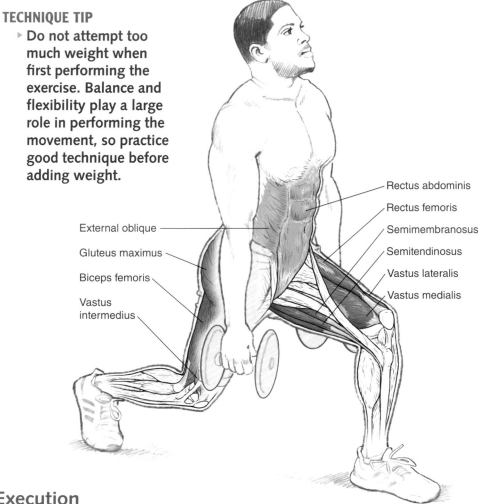

External oblique

Gluteus maximus

Biceps femoris

Vastus intermedius

Rectus abdominis

Rectus femoris

Semimembranosus

Semitendinosus

Vastus lateralis

Vastus medialis

Execution

1. Stand with legs shoulder-width apart, with good posture. Each hand is holding a dumbbell that is relatively light.
2. Take a small step forward with one leg, lowering your hips as you step so that your quadriceps are parallel to the ground and your lower leg is at a 90-degree angle at the knee. Your rear leg provides balance.
3. Return to the original position by pushing upward, after reaching parallel, with the same leg that made the initial step. Repeat the exercise for a full set of reps on one leg, or switch legs after a rep with each leg.

Muscles Involved

Primary: quadriceps, hamstrings, gluteus maximus

Secondary: rectus abdominis, external oblique

⚠ **SAFETY TIP** One caution for this exercise is to not allow the kneecap to extend past the toes of the lead foot while performing the movement. The possibility of injuring the knee because of its relatively vulnerable, unstable position while performing a difficult, anaerobic exercise is real. This is a wise rule to follow for most people; however, in a few runners with longer femurs, it is difficult not to extend past the toes. Practice the exercise in front of a mirror, and if your form is spot-on and your knees extend past your toes, so be it.

Running Focus

The lunge is a difficult exercise to master quickly. Like the squat, a similar movement, it develops strength throughout the core, hamstrings, and quadriceps, but mastering the proper form is difficult. It is important to master the technique before adding weight. A barbell instead of dumbbells can be used, but holding the barbell on the shoulders is an unnatural hand position for a runner. Keeping the hands low while holding the dumbbells is normally more comfortable for runners.

This exercise fits nicely in the second, or strength (threshold), phase of training. It is functional and, with the added weight of the dumbbells, can develop significant strength.

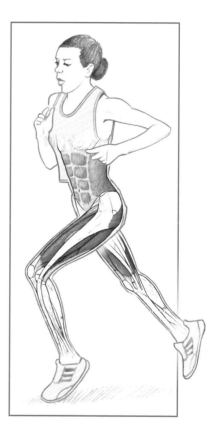

VARIATION

Lunge With Long Step

By taking a longer step, the gluteus medius and gluteus maximus of the leg that is forward are strengthened more than with a regular step, and the iliopsoas and rectus femoris of the back leg are stretched.

Machine Incline Leg Press

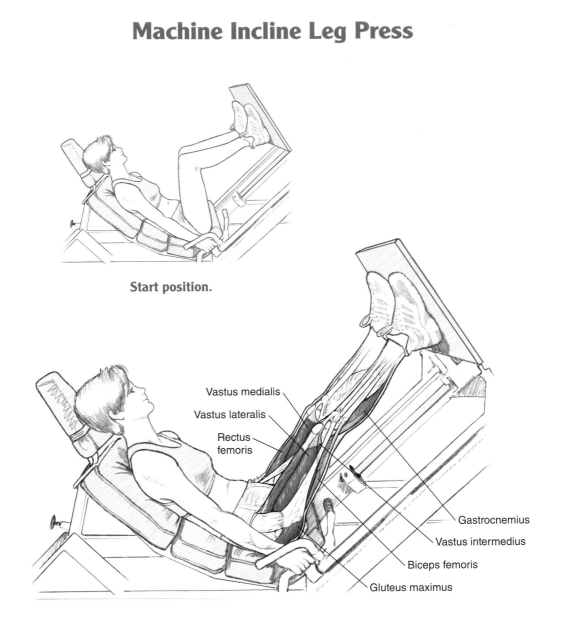

Start position.

Vastus medialis
Vastus lateralis
Rectus femoris
Gastrocnemius
Vastus intermedius
Biceps femoris
Gluteus maximus

Execution

1. Sit with the feet placed close together (narrower than shoulder-width apart) on the bottom part of the footplate. The back and the head are pressed against the back pads. The safety catch should be on. Flip the safety outward, rendering the weight active. The legs should be prepared to support the weight before the safety is released. Inhale.

2. Concentrating on the hips, glutes, and quads, extend the legs in a fluid movement to full extension by extending both knees.

3. Return to the starting position by gradually flexing the knees, allowing the weight to slowly lower back to the original position.

Muscles Involved

Primary: quadriceps, gluteus maximus

Secondary: gastrocnemius, biceps femoris

⚠️**SAFETY TIP** This exercise allows for a greater weight to be used because of its reliance on a machine; however, be careful not to add too much weight until proper form is established.

TECHNIQUE TIP
> Do not hurry the movement, which results in the weight moving past the full range of motion and bouncing back to the legs.

Running Focus

The machine incline leg press is a safe exercise to perform, and it can increase strength in the quadriceps and glutes quickly because relatively heavy weights can be used because of the incorporation of the machine. Instead of using energy and strength by heavily incorporating stabilizing muscles (abdominals and adductors), the exercise effectively isolates the quads and glutes, strengthening both sides of the upper leg, helping to avoid muscle imbalances and potential injury.

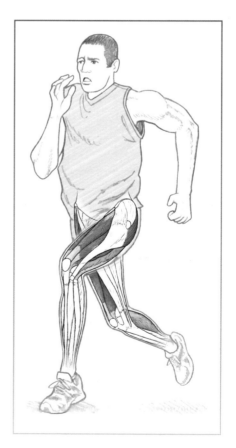

Altering foot position on the footplate will change the muscle groups impacted. To incorporate more of the glutes, place your feet at the top of the footplate.

Due to its emphasis on the large muscle groups, this exercise creates explosive power for runners. Therefore, it is best used by runners training for shorter events such as a 5K or for track racing in sprints or middle-distance events. The exercise is suitable during the introductory phase of training for all runners because it is a general strength exercise, not a functionally-specific strength exercise.

Bent-Leg Good Morning

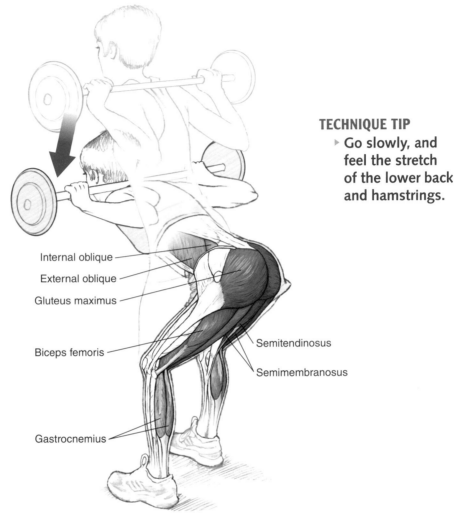

TECHNIQUE TIP
▸ Go slowly, and feel the stretch of the lower back and hamstrings.

Internal oblique

External oblique

Gluteus maximus

Biceps femoris

Semitendinosus

Semimembranosus

Gastrocnemius

Execution

1. Stand with good posture, feet shoulder-width apart, grasping a barbell of light weight across the shoulders.
2. Lower the torso by bowing at the waist. The back should be lowered in a single plane, maintaining the lumbar (lower back) curvature. The glutes push outward during the motion. Inhale during the downward movement.
3. Return to the standing position by raising the torso, focusing on the rotation of the pelvis.

Muscles Involved

Primary: hamstrings, gluteus maximus

Secondary: gastrocnemius, external oblique, internal oblique

Running Focus

Many distance runners complain that they feel chronic tightness in the lower back because of the accumulated mileage they have run in training. The jarring impact of a heel strike plus a lack of flexibility has caused many a runner to discontinue training and find another sport. How can you alleviate such a problem? Exercises like the bent-leg good morning, which actually strengthens and stretches the hamstrings in one exercise, work well. Again, like most of the exercises in this book, the bent-leg good morning is a simple exercise to perform, and it has multiple benefits. Aside from strengthening the hamstrings and glutes, it also helps stretch these muscles, helping to loosen the connective tissue between the muscles and the bones of the lower back and the pelvis. This kinetic chain also affects the knees because a more supple lower back pulls less on the hamstrings, in turn allowing the kneecaps to track normally.

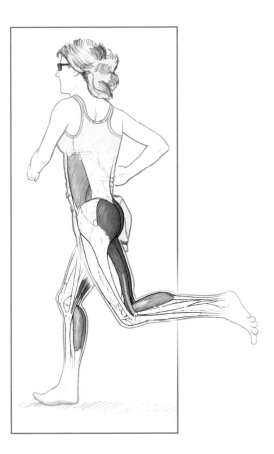

VARIATION

Straight-Leg Good Morning

The good morning can be performed with straight legs, but runners with chronically tight hamstrings should perform the exercise with bent legs because of the emphasis on hamstring flexibility. Once greater flexibility is attained, the straight-leg version can be incorporated.

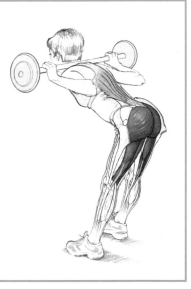

Dumbbell Romanian Deadlift

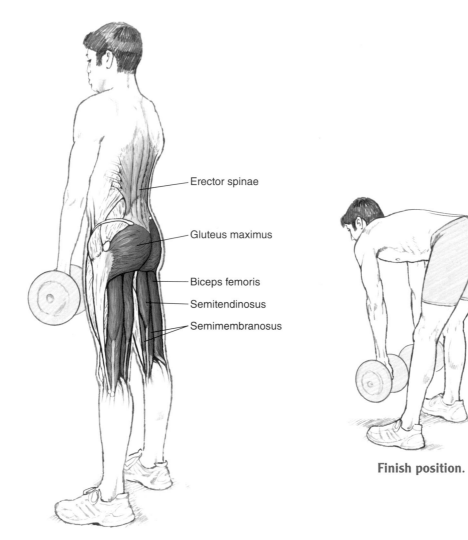

- Erector spinae
- Gluteus maximus
- Biceps femoris
- Semitendinosus
- Semimembranosus

Finish position.

Execution

1. Stand with feet slightly apart and legs slightly bent, with each arm extended downward holding a dumbbell with an overhand grip. There is a slight natural curve in the lower back.

2. Gradually bend at the waist, lowering your back in a single plane while maintaining the natural curve in the back, with the dumbbells almost scraping the quads and knees as you bend.

3. Return to the upright position once you can no longer lower the weight.

Muscles Involved

Primary: hamstrings, gluteus maximus

Secondary: erector spinae

TECHNIQUE TIP
▶ **The dumbbells should not reach the floor. The slight curve in the lower back should prevent that much movement.**

Running Focus

This intense exercise emphasizes the upper legs, specifically the hamstrings and glutes. It is extremely functional in that it works the muscles the way they work when running, more so than the hamstring curl. As has been noted previously, the balance between the larger quadriceps group and the hamstrings is the key to extension and propulsion during the gait cycle. To ensure uninterrupted training, avoidance of injury can be almost guaranteed by performing exercises like the dumbbell Romanian deadlift that help stretch and strengthen the back of the upper legs.

Also, given the demands of fast-paced running on the hamstrings, fast-twitch muscle fibers of the hamstrings are best trained with higher-intensity exercises like the dumbbell Romanian deadlift.

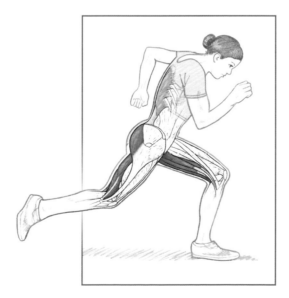

Squat

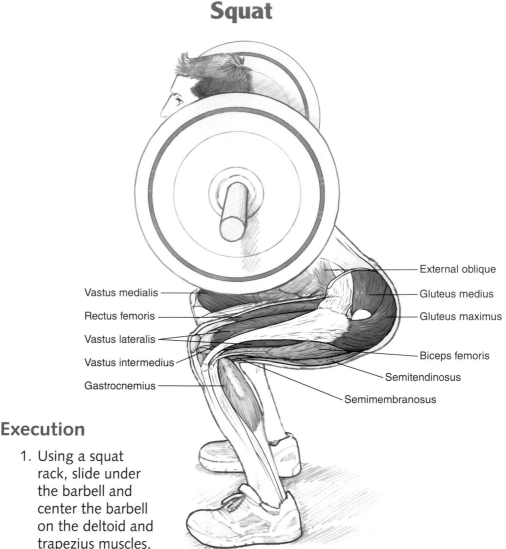

Vastus medialis
Rectus femoris
Vastus lateralis
Vastus intermedius
Gastrocnemius

External oblique
Gluteus medius
Gluteus maximus
Biceps femoris
Semitendinosus
Semimembranosus

Execution

1. Using a squat rack, slide under the barbell and center the barbell on the deltoid and trapezius muscles, not the vertebrae of the neck. Feet should be shoulder-width apart and splayed slightly.

2. Inhale deeply, expanding the chest. Maintain the natural curve in the lower back while straightening up and lifting the barbell off the rack.

3. Establish proper position by taking a few steps backward, repositioning the feet and reestablishing the accentuated curve in the lower back.

4. Look toward a point above head level, and initiate the squat action by bending forward at the hips, which will lower the rear. When the thighs are parallel to the floor, straighten the legs and return to the initial position while exhaling.

Muscles Involved

Primary: quadriceps, gluteus maximus, gluteus medius, gluteus minimus

Secondary: hamstrings, external oblique, gastrocnemius

Running Focus

The squat is primarily a quadriceps exercise, but because of its stability demand, it also helps strengthen the core, hamstrings, and muscles of the lower leg. Heavy weight can be lifted, but it is not necessary to make this exercise effective. Squats should be performed during the same session as the dumbbell Romanian deadlift or the good morning to create balance between the front and back of the legs.

Like the machine incline leg press, the squat creates explosive power due to its emphasis on the large muscle groups. Therefore, it is best suited for runners training for shorter events such as the 5K or for track racing in the sprints or middle distance events. Because it is a general strength exercise, not a functionally-specific strength exercise, it is suitable during the introductory phase for all runners. Its emphasis on core stability can aid all runners at every phase of the training progression.

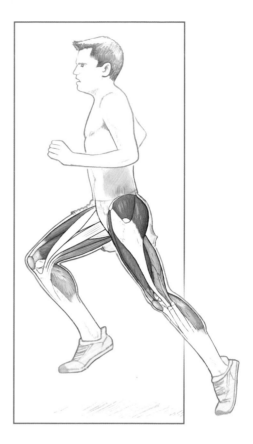

VARIATION

Single-Leg Squat With Dumbbells

This exercise aids in developing the adductor muscles of the inner thigh. Stand about two to three feet in front of a bench with a dumbbell in each hand. Place the top of one foot (laces of the shoe down) on the bench behind you. Lower your body until the forward leg is bent 90 degrees at the knee and the knee of the rear leg is almost touching the ground. Push back up using the quadriceps muscles of the forward leg. After performing a set of 12 on one leg, switch legs. The weight of the dumbbells does not need to be heavy. Initially, until good form is established, no added weight is necessary.

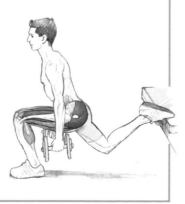

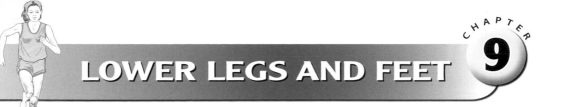
Any structure that will pass the test of longevity must have a strong, secure, and preferably wide base. The human being is certainly not a pyramid, which is the perfect example of such a design, yet to remain upright the human has to survive with two stable lower limbs, augmented by relatively large feet, over a fairly narrow base.

The tibia (figure 9.1) is the major weight-bearing bone of the lower leg. It is splinted by the thinner fibula, which becomes more relevant at the ankle, where it forms the outer part of this hinged and curved joint. The muscles attached to these bones control the movement of both the

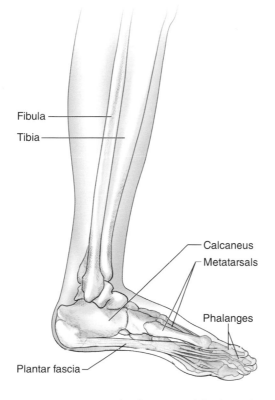

Figure 9.1 Bony structures and soft tissues of the lower leg and foot.

ankle and the metatarsals and phalanges that form the foot. The ankle joint itself moves almost entirely in the anterior-to-posterior plane, but the seven bones that form the tarsus are placed so that there can be both inversion and eversion of the foot at the midtarsal and subtalar joints. This allows each foot to turn inward and outward to accommodate for uneven or slippery ground underfoot.

Only three bones on the undersurface of the foot make contact with the ground. Under the heel is the calcaneum, and the first and fifth metatarsal heads complete the triangle. Between this tripod of bones is a complex consisting of the talus, cuboid, navicular, and three cuneiform bones, which lie in opposition to each other in such a way that they can be raised to form a longitudinal, or lengthwise, arch to each foot with the five metatarsal bones. Not only do they have to change position to compensate for variations underfoot, but they also allow the feet sideways movement. The tarsal bones form the apex of a bony arch, and when viewed from the ends of the toes appear to rotate on each other to enable the feet to move in or out. It is by this movement that walking or running on the inside or outside of the feet is possible.

The power from the calves to push forward comes from the two muscles of the posterior compartment (figure 9.2). The soleus is the deeper muscle and combines with the gastrocnemius to form the Achilles tendon, which is inserted into the calcaneum. Their contraction pulls this bone and thus the whole foot backward. A deeper layer of muscles provides flexion to the metatarsals and toes. These are the flexor digitorum longus, flexor hallucis longus, and tibialis posterior. They provide plantarflexion to the foot and, because they cross several joints, to the ankle as well.

The anterior, or extensor, compartment of the leg lies between the tibia and fibula and is surrounded by a relatively inelastic fibrous sheath. Within it are contained the tibialis anterior, extensor digitorum longus, and extensor hallucis longus muscles. These pass through the front of the ankle and are inserted into the tarsal, metatarsal, and toe bones in order to raise them or lift them up, an action known as dorsiflexion. These do not have to generate the same power as the posterior calf muscles for most activities, so they are less developed and weaker. Further lateral stability to the ankle and rear foot is provided by the peroneal muscles, which arise from the fibula and pass around the lateral side of the ankle joint to be inserted into the outer metatarsals.

Very powerful forces are generated through the Achilles tendon. If it is injured, it tends to be very painful because of its well-developed nerve supply and heals slowly because of poor blood flow. Much the same can be said of the plantar tendon, or fascia, which spreads from the front of the calcaneum and is inserted at the bases of the five metatarsals. It is an unyielding sheet of fibrous tissue whose weakest point is at the heel. If the foot is viewed two-dimensionally from the inside, the plantar tendon provides the horizontal base to the triangle completed by the tarsal and metatarsal bones.

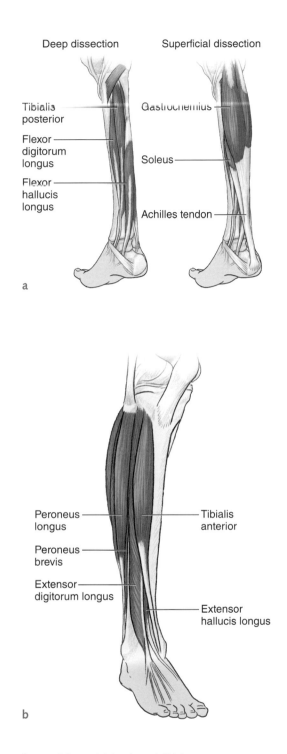

Deep dissection   Superficial dissection

Tibialis posterior

Gastrocnemius

Flexor digitorum longus

Soleus

Flexor hallucis longus

Achilles tendon

a

Peroneus longus

Tibialis anterior

Peroneus brevis

Extensor digitorum longus

Extensor hallucis longus

b

Figure 9.2   Lower leg and foot: *(a)* back and *(b)* front.

This anatomy must be considered on a functional basis, and watching a slow-motion recording of a foot landing and taking off is invaluable in understanding the motion involved in each stride. The initial plant of the foot is known as the heel strike, after which the foot turns a little inward, with the weight of the body progressively passing down the outer side of the foot before landing is completed on the ball formed by the metatarsal bases. Fewer runners meet the ground first with their toes, sometimes because of an inability to dorsiflex sufficiently. This lack of heel strike may be due to genetic or structural causes. Most people can run on their toes only for a very short time and distance because the work of plantarflexion is taken over by the comparatively weak toe flexors rather than the powerful calf muscles working through the pivot of the calcaneum, especially if dorsiflexion is limited.

Once the foot is flat, the movement continues in reverse; during take-off, the heel lifts off first, rolls inward along the outer metatarsals, and ends with the final push-off from the ball of the foot. During this action, all the muscles will contract or expand in a regular rhythm, though not at the same time.

At this juncture we need to demystify the superstitions that have developed around feet that are pronated or supinated. There are three related but separate elements to movement within the foot. At the sub-talar joint, the foot inverts and everts, or turns inwardly or outwardly. At the midfoot, there is abduction or adduction, where the movement is solely in the horizontal plane, while at the forefoot, the movement is principally up and down, in dorsiflexion, which somewhat confusingly describes an extension of the foot, or plantarflexion. Pronation describes a compound movement of these joints, where there is eversion at the subtalar joint, abduction (i.e., outward horizontal movement) at the midfoot, and dorsiflexion at the forefoot. Supination describes the opposite movement of each joint. Every foot, with every stride, exhibits some of these actions. When they become excessive, the runner may have difficulties that lead to pain or injury. Excessive pronation when the foot is flat on the ground, where the longitudinal arch of the foot leans excessively inward and the toes point outward, will stress the tibia by internally rotating it and the ligaments between the bones of the midfoot by stretching them, affecting the ability of the inverting muscles of the feet to perform efficiently. Supination describes the opposite action, in which the outside of the runner's foot takes the weight of landing on the ground. The tibia is disproportionately externally rotated, and the effect of the extra strain on the peroneal muscles may also spread to the iliotibial band. (In chapter 11 we demonstrate how appropriate footwear may minimize the distress that overpronation and supination may pose to the serious runner.) Because of the strains imposed when the feet are excessively overmobile, a severely supinated foot may prove too much of a handicap for a distance runner, though many of the fastest runners in the world have overcome this potential disability.

Another anatomical variation concerns those with high, rigid, longitudinal arches, who may also but not necessarily supinate, and those with flat arches with or without excessive pronation. For both of these types of feet, the lack of flexibility is likely to lead to a mechanical disadvantage in that they may be slower runners than they otherwise might.

Specific Training Guidelines

Some of the standing exercises are performed or can be performed unilaterally, meaning one leg at a time. This type of movement can significantly strengthen the targeted muscles by recruiting all the major leg muscles, weaker ones included, to establish balance while properly performing each exercise.

As mentioned in chapter 5 and thoroughly examined in chapter 7, exercises that require stability engage the core muscles of the abdomen, lower back, and hips to maintain proper form. Performing most freestanding exercises unilaterally helps ensure that the specific muscles targeted plus the core muscles recruited develop strength and, with enough reps, muscular endurance.

Single-Leg Heel Raise With Dumbbells

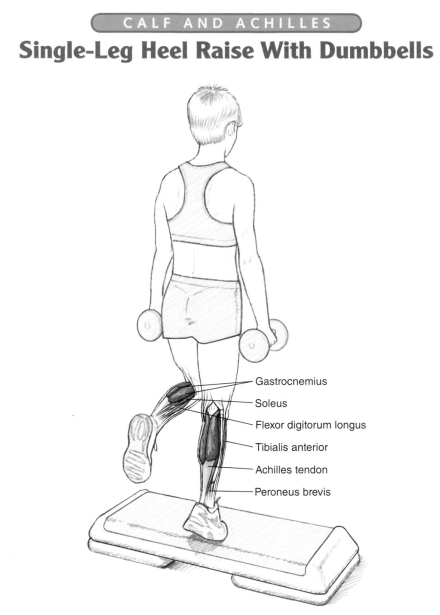

- Gastrocnemius
- Soleus
- Flexor digitorum longus
- Tibialis anterior
- Achilles tendon
- Peroneus brevis

Execution

1. Stand on a platform with one foot touching the platform with only the ball of the foot and the toes. The midfoot and the heel are not touching the platform. Hold the other leg at a 90-degree angle at the knee, from the hip, not touching the platform. Both hands should be holding dumbbells, with the arms extending straight down along the hips and sides of the quadriceps.

2. Maintaining proper posture, an erect upper body stabilized by the engagement of the abdominal muscles, rise up (plantarflexion) on the foot on the platform. Do not hyperextend the knee. The leg should be straight or slightly bent at approximately 5 degrees.

3. Lower the foot (dorsiflexion) back to the beginning position. Complete to tolerance each set and then repeat the exercise using the other leg.

Muscles Involved

Primary: gastrocnemius, soleus

Secondary: tibialis anterior, peroneus brevis, flexor digitorum longus

Soft Tissue Involved

Primary: Achilles tendon

TECHNIQUE TIP

▸ **The exercise should be performed until the calf muscles begin to burn. Do not perform to fatigue unless performing only one set. One to three sets will suffice, with the amount of weight held being a variable that can change the effect of the workout.**

Running Focus

The single-leg heel raise exercise should be a staple of every runner's strength-training regimen because it is a simply-performed exercise with very little equipment, and because it is a multipurpose exercise. Specifically, it can be performed to develop strength, which aids in injury prevention, and it can be used as a rehabilitation exercise if the Achilles tendon or calf muscles have been injured. The exercise should not be performed if a runner is still suffering the initial effects of the injury, but can be safely performed after the onset of the injury if some healing, determined by a subjective evaluation of the pain level or the evaluation of an objective image (MRI), has taken place.

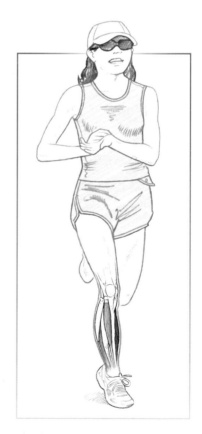

As described in chapter 10, adding an eccentric, or negative, component of the exercise (lengthening of the muscle) adds value to this specific calf and Achilles tendon exercise. Eccentric motions have value because the muscle can handle a lot more weight eccentrically contracting. It is also hypothesized that muscle strengthening is greatest when performing eccentric-contraction movements and that eccentric contractions are better suited to develop a muscle's fast-twitch fibers.

CALF AND ACHILLES
Machine Standing Heel Raise

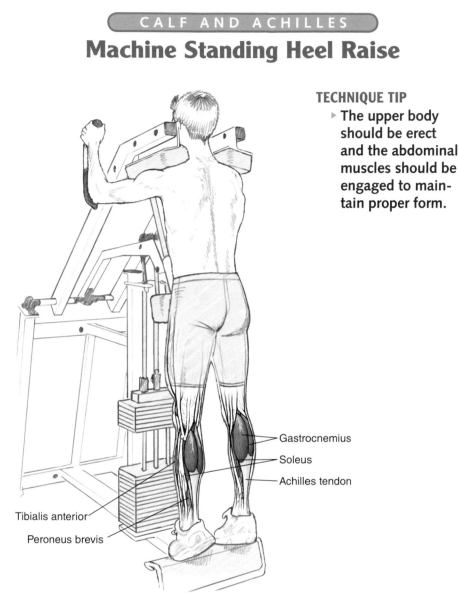

TECHNIQUE TIP
▸ **The upper body should be erect and the abdominal muscles should be engaged to maintain proper form.**

Gastrocnemius
Soleus
Achilles tendon
Tibialis anterior
Peroneus brevis

Execution

1. Stand under the shoulder pads of the machine so that there is a small amount of flex at the knees. The upper body should be erect and the abdominal muscles should be engaged to maintain proper form. Arms should be placed on the handles next to the shoulder pads. A light grip should be used.

2. Elevate the heels (plantarflexion) until both feet are only touching the platform with the metatarsals and toes; however, the toes should be relaxed and the emphasis should be on the extension of the calf muscles.

3. Lower the heels until a full stretch of the calves is felt. Repeat.

Muscles Involved

Primary: gastrocnemius, soleus

Secondary: tibialis anterior, peroneus brevis

Soft Tissue Involved

Primary: Achilles tendon

Running Focus

The standing heel raise is another exercise designed to strengthen the complex of calf muscles (gastrocnemius and soleus) and the Achilles tendon. Its emphasis is more on the gastrocnemius, the larger portion of the calf, than the soleus, but it does work the smaller muscle also. This exercise can be done during the same workout as the single-leg heel raise to really fatigue the calf muscles, or it can be done independently of the other exercises when the goal of the workout is to perform one exercise per body part.

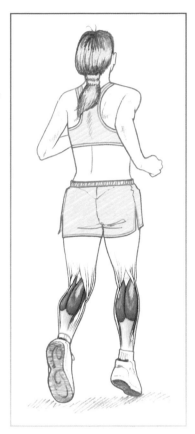

The Achilles tendon and calf muscles take on much of the shock absorption and deflection after heel strike. When a runner races in lightweight shoes with a lower heel height than traditional trainers, the impact becomes more pronounced. To help minimize impact and aid in propulsion by moving the foot through its cycle, all runners should include exercises to develop calf strength in their training. These exercises can be performed during any stage of the running progression, with special emphasis during the racing phase if no injury has occurred.

VARIATION

Machine Seated Heel Raise

Similarities between the anatomy affected by the standing heel raise and seated heel raise abound, but it is the emphasis on the soleus muscle that differentiates the two exercises. When sitting, the gastrocnemius muscle is less involved in the exercise, allowing the soleus, despite its smaller size, to become the dominant calf muscle.

The strengthening of the soleus aids in the propulsive force of the takeoff phase of the running gait cycle. It also aids the runner who races (or works out) in racing flats to overcome calf pain and Achilles tendon strain during and following a race or a workout. The lower heel height of the flat or spike forces the Achilles tendon to stretch more than in running shoes. A strengthened and stretched soleus muscle helps prevent injury to the Achilles tendon by mitigating the extra stretch.

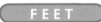

Plantarflexion With Tubing

Calcaneofibular
ligament

Tibialis posterior

Flexor hallucis longus

Execution

1. Sit on the floor with legs fully extended in front of the body. A length of surgical tubing, an end in each hand, should extend underneath the foot, wrapping around the ball of the foot where the metatarsal heads are located. The tubing needs to be taut, with no slack, before the exercise begins.

2. Extend (plantarflex) the foot to full extension.

3. At full extension, hold the position for one second before pulling the tubing backward in a smooth, continuous fashion. The foot will be forced to dorsiflex and return to its initial position.

4. Repeat the push and pull of the exercise, adjusting tension throughout, until fatigue.

Muscles Involved

Primary: tibialis posterior, flexor hallucis longus

Soft Tissue Involved

Primary: posterior talofibular ligament, calcaneofibular ligament

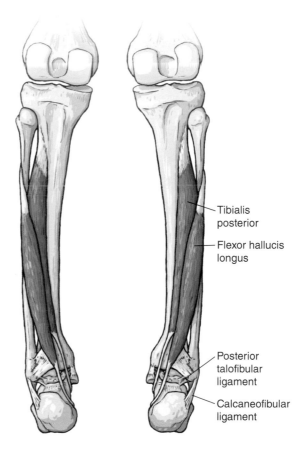

Tibialis posterior

Flexor hallucis longus

Posterior talofibular ligament

Calcaneofibular ligament

Running Focus

In chapter 4, a discussion of the adaptations required for running at different speeds and terrains offers some insight into the role of the feet and ankles in running performance. This exercise promotes strength and flexibility of the foot and ankle to prevent injury when running on uneven terrain and aids in the support phase of the gait cycle.

Because this exercise is not weight bearing, it can be performed daily. It can function as a rehabilitative exercise to overcome an ankle sprain, or it can stand alone as a strengthening exercise to promote improved strength and flexibility. Because the exerciser controls the tension of the surgical tubing, the exercise can be made as difficult or as easy as possible for each repetition. The emphasis should be on a smooth but explosive movement with the appropriate resistance being provided by the tautness of the tubing, which can easily be adjusted by applying or lessening tension through gradually pulling or releasing the ends of the tubing held in each hand.

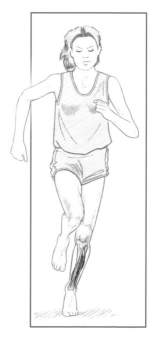

FEET

Dorsiflexion With Ankle Weights

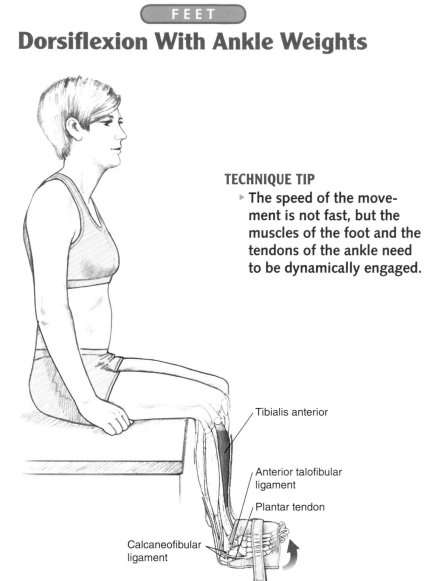

TECHNIQUE TIP
> The speed of the move-
> ment is not fast, but the
> muscles of the foot and the
> tendons of the ankle need
> to be dynamically engaged.

Tibialis anterior

Anterior talofibular
ligament

Plantar tendon

Calcaneofibular
ligament

Execution

1. Sit on a table with knees bent and lower legs dangling. An ankle weight providing appropriate resistance is secured around the mid-foot. The upper body is erect with hands by the sides providing balance only.

2. In a smooth but forceful motion, the foot dorsiflexes (points upward and back) toward the tibia to full extension. The lower leg remains bent at 90 degrees and does not swing to aid the foot and ankle in moving the weight.

3. Gently lower (plantarflex) the foot (it does not need to be fully extended) and repeat the exercise to fatigue. Switch the ankle weight to the other foot and repeat the exercise.

Muscles Involved

Primary: tibialis anterior

Soft Tissue Involved

Primary: anterior talofibular ligament, calcaneofibular ligament, plantar tendon

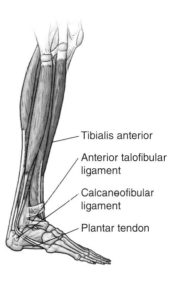

Tibialis anterior

Anterior talofibular ligament

Calcaneofibular ligament

Plantar tendon

Running Focus

This is another non-weight-bearing foot and ankle exercise that can be done daily both as an injury rehabilitation exercise as well as to improve strength and flexibility. The amount of weight of the ankle cuff can be varied to fine-tune the goal of the exercise. For example, a heavier weight performed fewer times with fewer sets emphasizes the strengthening of the anatomy affected. A lighter weight allows for more repetitions and sets, which aids the flexibility and endurance of the anatomy affected.

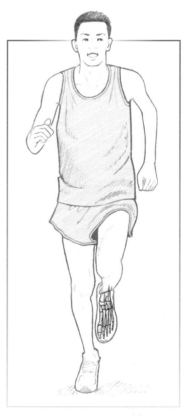

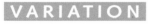

Dorsiflexion With Tubing

This exercise can also be done with tubing, like the plantarflexion exercise. It can actually be done alternately by first plantarflexing the foot against the resistance of the tubing, and then immediately resisting when the tubing is pulled toward the body, until it is fully flexed and ready to plantarflex again.

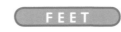

Foot Eversion With Elastic Band

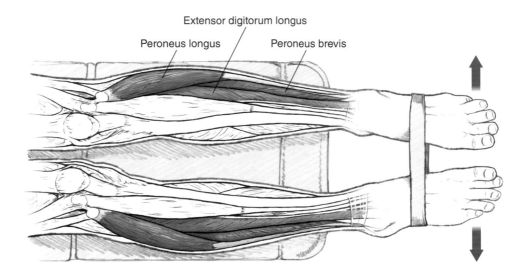

Extensor digitorum longus

Peroneus longus

Peroneus brevis

Execution

1. Sit on a weight bench with the legs fully extended so that only the Achilles tendons, ankles, and feet are off the bench. Support the body by placing both hands on the bench behind the body. Wrap an elastic band tautly around both feet, which are plantarflexed, soles down, leaving approximately six inches of space between the feet.

2. Rotate the feet inward, dropping the big toes, and pushing outward with the feet against the resistance of the band. Hold for three to five seconds.

3. Relax the feet, rest for three to five seconds, and repeat.

Muscles Involved

Primary: peroneus longus, peroneus brevis, extensor digitorum longus

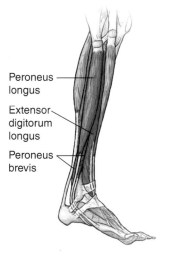

Peroneus longus

Extensor digitorum longus

Peroneus brevis

Running Focus

As mentioned in the introduction to this chapter, pronation happens as a result of movements on three planes, not just one. One of these movements is the eversion of the foot; during plantarflexion, eversion is controlled mainly by the peroneus longus, and in dorsiflexion, the peroneus brevis. This exercise is performed in the plantarflexed position because it is an easier movement, particularly for a runner who is an overpronator. Underpronators, also called supinators, benefit from this exercise because it is not the natural motion of their feet.

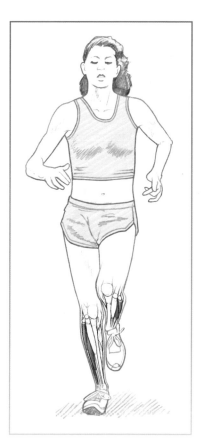

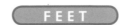

Foot Inversion on Bosu Ball

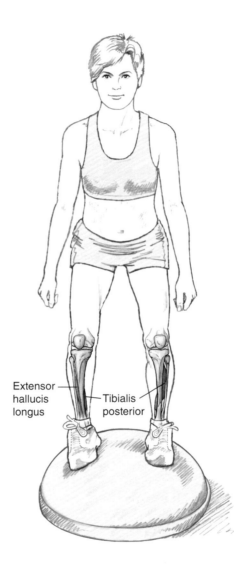

Extensor
hallucis
longus

Tibialis
posterior

Execution

1. Step onto a properly inflated Bosu ball with the dome side up. Establish foot position to ensure a properly balanced body.

2. While standing on the Bosu ball with feet in an inverted position, perform any standing exercise from the book (see the Running Focus section that follows for details).

3. Fatigue sets in quickly, so stepping onto a flat surface as a break between reps on the Bosu ball can be taken as needed.

Muscles Involved

Primary: tibialis posterior

Secondary: extensor hallucis longus

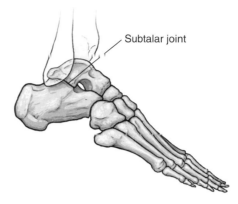

Subtalar joint

Running Focus

Bosu balls are touted by fitness trainers as a tool for developing balance and proprioception. The development of balance and proprioception benefits the runner racing and training off-road, and the improved ankle strength and flexibility derived from the inverted position of each foot on the ball supports each foot through the gait cycle. The exercise performed is less important than the emphasis placed on maintaining balance on the Bosu ball. Given the curvature of the dome, the feet are in an inverted position on the ball throughout the exercise. For example, performing squats with dumbbells would be a good exercise to promote strengthening of the feet and ankles in the inverted position. Another less dynamic exercise would be to perform dumbbell curls. Or you could do one set or multiple sets of each. The emphasis is on the inverted position of the foot, but combining it with another exercise makes for a time-saving compound movement.

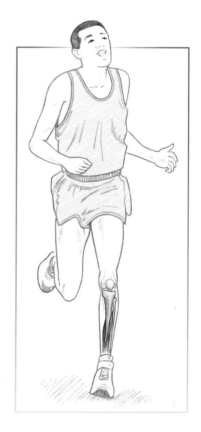

The use of the Bosu ball also adds a twist to normal strength-training exercises like dumbbell curls and dumbbell squats, making for a more varied and enjoyable strength-training routine. However, some exercises should not be performed on the Bosu ball. Specifically, exercises that require placing a lot of weight and torque on the knee joints (e.g., full squats with heavy weight) should be avoided.

COMMON RUNNING INJURIES

I f this book had been written without thought for any downside to running, we would have done readers a great disservice. It would be naive in the extreme to imagine that it is possible to run and exercise in a more efficient manner without meeting some of the pitfalls that almost every runner encounters at some time. Some of these are beyond human control, but others are certainly preventable if thought is given to the long-term aim of the training program.

If the exercises in this book are followed, the time allocated both to exercise and to running will increase. One handy rule is never to step up either the mileage or the time spent running by more than 5 to 10 percent per week. This cannot apply in the initial stages of a training schedule, where less than 10 miles a week are run, but above these levels, this guide will help to prevent overuse injuries. Pain is probably the best warning sign of injury, but it may appear in a variety of forms. Although the suffering that occurs during a tough training session is probably ultimately beneficial in the improvement of performance, the experienced runner will soon learn to recognize pain in other parts of the anatomy that does not disappear when the exercise has ended.

External factors that may induce injury include the surface run on and the clothing and shoes worn by the runner. The force of landing with something like three to four times your body weight onto concrete affects the joints much more than a more forgiving and softer surface like sand or even snow. Too many runners use only one side of a road and forget that the camber will pitch them toward the sidewalk and cause a tilt to the pelvis, which may translate into a twisted lower back or strain to the ligaments of the ankle joint. Running demands thought just as much as other sports that require different skills. It is too easy to be dazzled by a new pair of running shoes, which cause blistering on the first occasion on which they are used, simply because you forgot to break them in. All shoes and clothing should be worn in but not worn out!

Because the diagnosis of injury is likely to be complex, any unexplained pain or symptom should be rapidly assessed by a professionally qualified doctor. However, a considerable number of commonsense first aid measures can and should be taken in the early stages of injury.

It would seem sensible to follow the guidelines that any doctor would use. First, take a history. Ask yourself these questions: Was the injury sudden, or did it build up over a series of runs? Does it cover a small area, or is it more diffuse? Does it hurt to touch? Does it disappear with rest? There are countless more questions, but the object is to make you think about the injury. Next, a doctor will look at the injury. Observation can distinguish asymmetry, swelling, discoloration, and so on. You can do the same in a mirror. Only this stage of examination by gentle palpation, followed by active and passive movement, will elucidate the cause. By this stage there may be a differential diagnosis, a choice of likely and then less common causes. If the diagnosis is pretty much certain, first aid treatment can begin; if not, further tests can be arranged after a visit to the doctor. To a certain extent these can run concurrently, as treatment can be started while test results are awaited. If the results suggest a different diagnosis, then treatment can be amended. The diagnosis and treatment phases of an injury should be interrelated and reciprocal so that if the one is questionable or ineffective, then the other can be reviewed and reassessed.

The areas of the body that are likely to suffer most from running are the lower back, the groin, the muscles of the leg, the knee and ankle areas, and the feet. The tissues that suffer most are joints, bones, ligaments, muscles, and tendons. Some choice!

A typical muscle tear is most likely to occur if the runner overstretches between two joints, especially if a halfhearted warm-up procedure has been used. The pathology behind this is that a blood vessel inside the muscle will be pulled beyond its limits, burst, relatively flood the area with blood, and stop bleeding only when the counterpressure exerted by the surrounding soft tissues or strapping is equal to that of the blood seeping out. The pressure of this bleeding causes pain in the soft tissues and is always a good indicator of injury. Cooling is another major factor that speeds up healing, so the rapid application of an ice pack to any acute injury, muscle or otherwise, is unlikely to do much harm; if it limits the swelling, it may well reduce the time spent in recovery.

Statistically, the back and the knee are the most commonly injured sites for runners. A runner's back pain will usually be localized to the lower lumbar and sacral areas (figure 10.1), and all too often it is a result of repetitive training with a lack or loss of low back flexibility, accompanied by attempts to run through the pain. It may be related to poor posture, a real or artificial difference in leg length (such as what occurs with the camber running referred to earlier), or a sudden move to hill work. If there is any suggestion that the pain is referred down either leg or is associated with numbness or weakness of the limb, then this could signify a more serious condition such as a prolapsed intervertebral disc, for which a more urgent medical opinion should be sought.

Much the same is true of the knee (figure 10.2). An injury followed by swelling or locking within the joint, especially if this happens rapidly over a few hours, is not a simple runner's knee and needs prompt diagnosis. Runners are more prone to patellofemoral pain as a result of the failure of the patella to glide through the center of the groove at the base of the femur rather than severe internal disruption as might occur with a skiing or football injury. When we stand, our knees and ankles are usually together, but the hip joints can be separated by 12 inches or more. The effect is that when the quadriceps muscles contract, the forces of nature pull the patella laterally and twist it within the femoral groove. The vastus medialis muscle counteracts the pull of the outer quads, but can do so only if it has been strengthened and developed suffi-

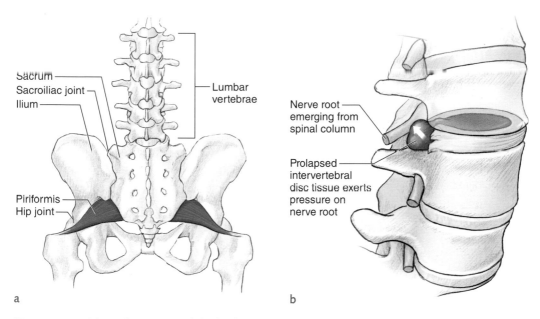

Sacrum
Sacroiliac joint
Ilium

Lumbar
vertebrae

Nerve root
emerging from
spinal column

Prolapsed
intervertebral
disc tissue exerts
pressure on
nerve root

Piriformis
Hip joint

a

b

Figure 10.1 *(a)* Lumbar region of the back; *(b)* vertebrae.

ciently, which requires it to be exercised with the knee locked and extended. If pain can be localized, it is easier to diagnose the cause. Pain on the outside of the lower thigh is in all probability a result of iliotibial band (ITB) syndrome, in which this piece of generally inelastic connective tissue rubs against the lateral condyle of the femur. If appropriate exercises to stretch it fail, podiatric adjustment of shoes and insoles may bring about a cure.

This treatment may also help with the foot pain of metatarsalgia. With a dropped longitudinal arch (known as pes planus, or flat feet), constant landing on a particular bone in the foot and a pull on the surrounding ligaments can be extremely painful, but proper support to the arch with exercises for the intrinsic muscles of the feet may dissipate the pain rapidly.

Pain associated with bones is deeper and more resistant to analgesia than that from the soft tissues. One particularly important cause of bone pain is the so-called stress fracture, which can be equated with metal fatigue or the crack that can occur in a china cup. (Figure 10.3 shows the most

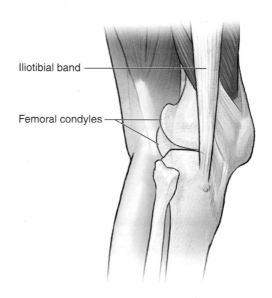

Iliotibial band

Femoral condyles

Figure 10.2 Knee.

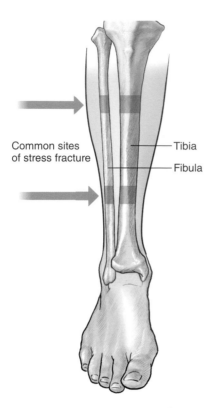

Common sites of stress fracture

Tibia

Fibula

Figure 10.3 Common sites of stress fractures in the tibia and fibula.

common sites of stress fractures in runners, in the tibia and fibula.) The fracture is undoubtedly present, but the opposing surfaces remain together because of surface tension and the binding from soft tissues. It is characterized by "crescendo" pain, which worsens with increasing distance run; it most commonly but not exclusively affects the lower leg or foot, and it stops only when the run finishes. On the next run it will begin earlier and worsen sooner. If this symptom is ignored, it may proceed to a complete fracture, with all the potential for disability of any broken bone, and will take at least double the time of a stress fracture to heal. Any runner with these symptoms who suspects a stress fracture is strongly advised to stop running immediately and seek a definitive diagnosis.

Plantar fasciitis is often such a painful condition that it commonly prevents any running at all. The weakest part of this sheet of fibrous tissue that runs between the heel and the metatarsal heads (figure 10.4) is at the heel, where it becomes injured through chronic overuse, ill-fitting shoes, or sudden stretching from an irregularity in the running surface. The typical sufferer will wince when the underside of the heel is even lightly touched. If the exercises in this chapter are ineffective, then a physician's steroid injection can produce a cure.

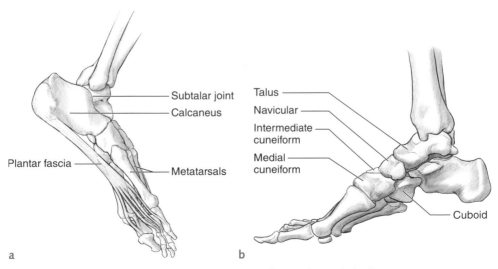

Subtalar joint

Calcaneus

Plantar fascia

Metatarsals

Talus

Navicular

Intermediate cuneiform

Medial cuneiform

Cuboid

a

b

Figure 10.4 Foot: *(a)* underside showing plantar fascia; *(b)* medial side.

If an Achilles (figure 10.5) or any other tendon is injured, healing is delayed by the poor blood supply to these tissues. Although the diagnosis may not be too difficult—the tendon becomes locally tender and stiff, especially if stretched—there has been much dispute concerning the best method of treatment. Current opinion tends toward a regimen of extensive stretching, which needs to be repeated endlessly even after a cure has been effected in an attempt to prevent recurrence. To be of value, a stretch should be uncomfortable rather than painful, held for between 15 to 30 seconds, and never used in a jerky or unstable position, such as the performance of a quadriceps stretch by standing on one leg.

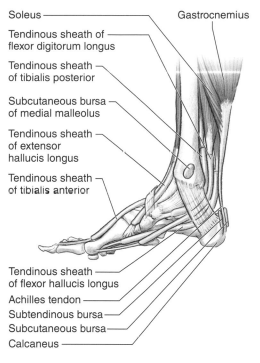

Soleus — Gastrocnemius

Tendinous sheath of flexor digitorum longus

Tendinous sheath of tibialis posterior

Subcutaneous bursa of medial malleolus

Tendinous sheath of extensor hallucis longus

Tendinous sheath of tibialis anterior

Tendinous sheath of flexor hallucis longus

Achilles tendon

Subtendinous bursa

Subcutaneous bursa

Calcaneus

Figure 10.5 Tendons, bones, and muscles of the lower leg and foot.

Note, however, that self-diagnosis of any sporting injury is fraught with danger. Every injury is different in some way from every other and each requires individual assessment and management. It would be irresponsible of us to attempt to manage injury in a book that is aimed at improvement, so the preceding paragraphs should encourage you, the runner, to be aware that your body is not just a mean, well-oiled speed machine but, like all machinery, may need a little fine-tuning!

Specific Training Guidelines

Warm up by doing some light running before performing the stretch. If the stretch is part of a rehabilitation of a tight iliotibial band and running is not an option, walk or perform a warm-up exercise for the legs for 10 minutes to promote blood flow.

There are many supposedly therapeutic treatments for running injuries, and many methods of performing those treatments. For example, the role of stretching in running training is widely debated. How often, what body parts to stretch, and how long to hold the stretch are some of the questions most runners ask running experts. Because the emphasis of this book is anatomy and strength training, an in-depth examination of these topics and the unraveling of the mysteries of stretching are left to you. We offer some best practices, but we also believe in the authorship of your own running training system. Attempt the strength-training and rehabilitation exercises prescribed in this book, and supplement these with others that your experience has proven successful.

ITB Stretch

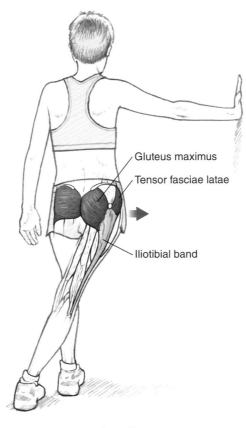

Gluteus maximus

Tensor fasciae latae

Iliotibial band

Standing.

Execution for Standing ITB Stretch

1. Stand next to a wall. Cross the outside leg in front of the inside leg (closest to the wall). Press a hand against the wall for support.

2. Lean the inside hip toward the wall, touching the wall if possible. Both feet should remain flat on the ground.

3. Hold the static stretch for 15 to 30 seconds. Repeat multiple times. Switch sides.

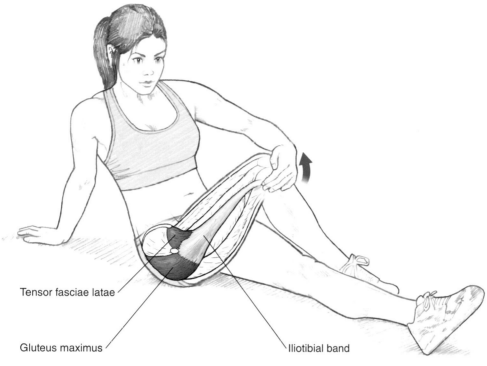

Tensor fasciae latae

Gluteus maximus

Iliotibial band

Sitting.

Execution for Sitting ITB Stretch

1. Sit on the floor with one leg extended and the other leg crossed at the knee, knee in the air, and foot firmly on the ground. The opposite hand is supporting the knee joint.
2. Gently press the outside of the knee that is crossed toward the opposite armpit.
3. Hold the static stretch for 15 to 30 seconds. Repeat multiple times. Switch sides.

Muscles Involved

Primary: gluteus maximus, tensor fasciae latae

Soft Tissue Involved

Primary: iliotibial band

Running Focus

As mentioned in chapter 9, tight iliotibial bands are normally a result of supination, not overpronation. The inversion of the foot can cause tight calves, lateral knee pain, and tight iliotibial bands. Even pronators who are overcorrected by their stability shoes or orthotics, essentially creating underpronation, can suffer from this injury. Performing the standing and sitting iliotibial band stretch will help stretch this thick band of soft tissue, preventing the painful rubbing over its attachment at the lateral femoral epicondyle. These stretches can be performed several times a day.

Proprioceptive Standing Balance

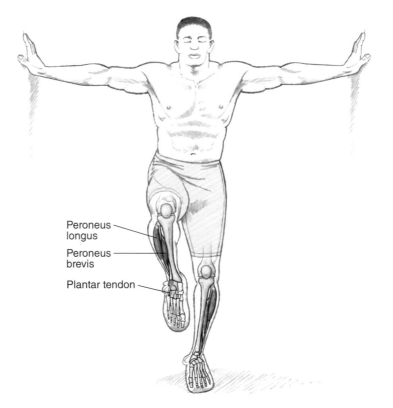

Peroneus longus

Peroneus brevis

Plantar tendon

Execution

1. Stand between two walls, one on each side. Extend the arms sideways at shoulder height for balance. Do not use the walls to balance unless needed to prevent falling.
2. Lift one knee until it is at a 90-degree angle with the hip and the tibia is at a 90-degree angle to the femur. Close your eyes.
3. Hold the position for 15 to 30 seconds. Lower the leg and repeat with the other leg. Perform multiple reps.

Muscles Involved

Primary: peroneus longus, peroneus brevis

Soft Tissue Involved

Primary: plantar tendon

Running Focus

This exercise has a neuromuscular and physiological component. It may take a while to establish proper balance, but the foot and lower leg are working to find equilibrium, so the exercise is productive even if you don't find balance immediately.

Standing Calf Stretch

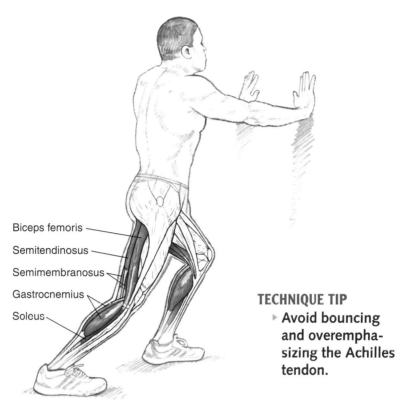

Biceps femoris
Semitendinosus
Semimembranosus
Gastrocnemius
Soleus

TECHNIQUE TIP
▸ **Avoid bouncing and overemphasizing the Achilles tendon.**

Execution

1. Stand, facing a wall with one leg extended backward, foot planted on the ground. The other leg, flexed at the knee, has the foot planted on the ground straight down from the hip. Arms are extended forward at upper-chest height, shoulder-width apart. Hands are placed on the wall.

2. Press gently into the wall and gradually press the heel of the extended leg into the floor. A stretch should be felt through the length of the gastrocnemius.

3. Stretch statically for 15 to 30 seconds and repeat multiple times, or switch legs after every rep.

Muscles Involved

Primary: gastrocnemius, soleus, hamstrings

Running Focus

Runners with neutral or underpronated biomechanics often suffer with tight calves. This stretch helps alleviate the pain of a chronically injured calf and also helps prevent calf injuries by keeping the muscle supple.

Standing Heel Raise With Eccentric Component

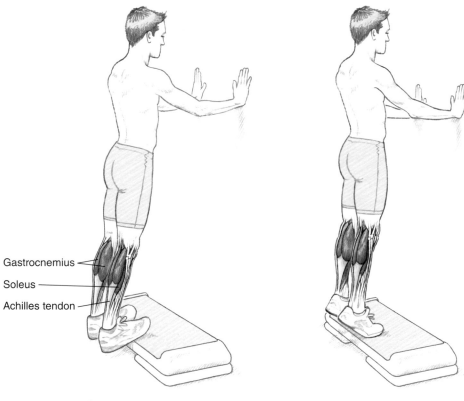

Start position.   Finish position.

Execution

1. Stand with both feet on a step with the heels off the step. Hands are pressed against the wall in front.
2. Raise up onto the metatarsal heads of both feet to full extension (plantarflexed).
3. Lower gradually to full extension (dorsiflexed).

Muscles Involved

Primary: gastrocnemius, soleus

Soft Tissue Involved

Primary: Achilles tendon

TECHNIQUE TIP
> ▸ Do not forcefully dorsiflex; it will place too much stress on the Achilles tendon.

Running Focus

This exercise both concentrically contracts (shortens) the calf muscle during plantarflexion and eccentrically contracts (lengthens) the muscle during dorsiflexion. As mentioned in chapter 9, including an eccentric, or negative, component adds value to this specific calf and Achilles tendon exercise. Studies have found that performing exercises with an eccentric component actually shortens the time it takes to heal an injury.

Hamstring Stretch

Execution

1. Sit upright lengthwise on a bench in a stable position. The leg with the hamstrings to be stretched is on the bench, and the other leg is placed on the floor with the foot flat to help stabilize the position. Place a towel or soft roll under the knee to be stretched with the knee bent no more than 5 degrees, and rest the heel lightly on the bench.

2. Move the torso forward toward the bench and flex at the hip joints to stretch the hamstrings. Maintain the position for 10 seconds or so, then slowly unwind. (There is no need to stretch out with the arms or to grasp the shin. This may lead to poor posture and an ineffective stretch!) Repeat three times. Alternate both legs in turn.

Muscles Involved

Primary: hamstrings

Secondary: piriformis

TECHNIQUE TIP

▸ There is no need to perform a hamstring stretch with the knee straight for specifically increasing hamstring muscle flexibility. When the leg is straightened, the tendency is for the stretch to be taken up more by the tendons and less by the hamstrings.

Running Focus

There are some runners whose particular style is to "pitter-patter" along with a short stride. Even if they are successful, this sort of running does them no favors if the race speeds up or a final sprint is involved. This exercise helps to increase the stride length without putting more strain on the lower back and sacroiliac regions. It should enable the stride length to be maintained longer as the runner tires, and eventually lead to improved performance.

Seated Knee Press

Execution

1. Sit upright in a comfortable position with room to extend the legs and knees. The back should be against a solid, supportive object. Both knees are slightly bent, heels on the floor.

2. Slowly straighten one knee in an attempt to push the back of that knee into the ground. Hold this position for six seconds.

3. Relax and allow the knee to flex slightly back to its resting position. Repeat the exercise but with the opposite leg. Do 10 repetitions with both knees.

Muscles Involved

Primary: vastus medialis

Secondary: rectus femoris, vastus lateralis, vastus intermedius, hamstrings, gastrocnemius

Soft Tissue Involved

Primary: posterior cruciate ligament, hip joint ligaments

TECHNIQUE TIP

▶ **If you perform this correctly, you should have a pulling sensation at the back of the knee, and a visible bulge will appear above and medial to the knee as the vastus medialis is contracted and its bulk develops.**

Running Focus

Knee pain is the greatest source of difficulty for most runners; runner's knee is the biggest culprit. This exercise strengthens the vastus medialis muscle and counteracts the slightly lateral (outward) pull of the other quadriceps muscles, which tends to cause patellofemoral pain as the bone shifts in the femoral groove. There is no nonoperative cure other than the development of the vastus medialis muscle, so this should be an essential exercise in every runner's training program.

Knee-to-Chest Stretch

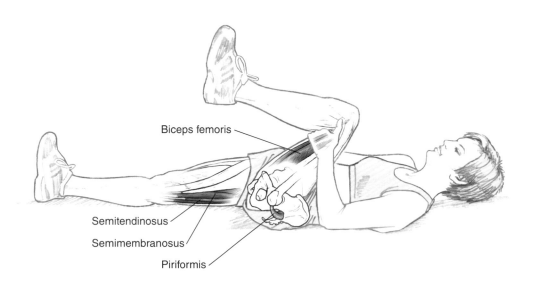

Biceps femoris

Semitendinosus

Semimembranosus

Piriformis

Execution

1. Lie on your back on a firm but comfortable surface.
2. Use the quadriceps to lift and bend the knee to 90 degrees, then grasp behind the knee with both hands and pull it toward the chest so that you feel a pulling sensation in the lowest part of the back and upper buttocks. At the same time, resist the urge to flex the other hip, but push it down onto the surface.
3. Hold the position for 15 to 30 seconds and repeat no more than five times, two or three times per day. Alternate with the other leg.

Muscles Involved

Primary: hamstrings

Secondary: piriformis, erector spinae

Running Focus

The lower back is usually ignored as a vital element of running until pain develops. By then it may be too late to correct. This exercise and those that follow give the lower back flexibility and strength. This is particularly important when climbing or descending hills. If the back can accommodate the changes of gradient, the stride length will also be increased by this flexibility in the hips and lower back. As with all stretching exercises, the aim should be to achieve discomfort without pain.

Wall Press

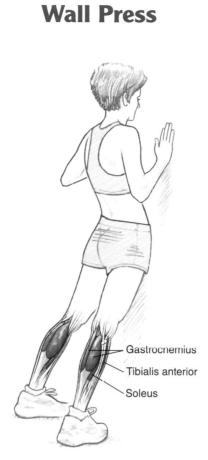

Gastrocnemius
Tibialis anterior
Soleus

Execution

1. Stand approximately 18 inches from a wall with feet shoulder-width apart, toes pointed inward.
2. Press your pelvis to the wall, adjusting the distance from the wall and the angle of the toes to gain the best stretch of the soleus. Keep your heels on the floor.
3. Hold stretch for 15 to 30 seconds and repeat.

Muscles Involved

Primary: soleus, gastrocnemius, tibialis anterior

Running Focus

Shin splints, or diffuse anterior lower leg pain, can be either soft-tissue related or bone (tibia) related. Both problems usually stem from overpronation; however, the soft-tissue variety is normally associated with midfoot horizontal plane abduction. This exercise can help prevent muscle pain in the anterior compartment of the gastrocnemius. This exercise can be performed multiple times daily and is effective when done regularly.

Ankle Plantarflexion

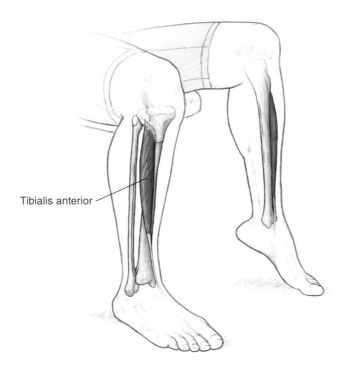

Tibialis anterior

Execution

1. Sit upright on a comfortable, hard-backed chair. The
   foot is initially flat on the
   floor, with the knee bent
   about 45 degrees or so,
   depending on the height
   of the chair. Raise the heel
   off the ground, then invert
   the foot as though pointing
   the toes like a ballet dancer.
   Hold the position for 15
   seconds and repeat up to
   10 times, two or three times
   per day, with both feet.

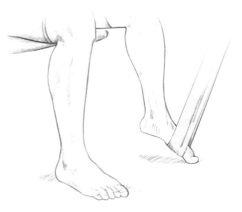

With tubing.

2. Place the chair in a position where a piece of flexible elastic such as
   Theraband can be attached to an immovable object on a wall in a
   loop. Sit in the same stretched position as previously and put the
   elastic around the midfoot farthest away from the wall. Use this as
   resistance to ease the foot farther into inversion and pull against it,
   strengthening the tibialis anterior muscle. Hold the position for 15
   seconds and repeat up to 10 times, two or three times per day, with
   both feet.

Muscles Involved

Primary: tibialis anterior

Running Focus

The importance of the tibialis anterior muscle is in the flexibility it gives to the ankles and feet. It is very involved in increasing stability when running on uneven terrain because it helps to adjust the position of the foot and therefore the leg. As such, any prolonged hill or undulating rough ground will bring it increasingly into use. If untrained, it will tire rapidly and slow the runner down, as well as increase the risk of a sprained ankle. When strengthened, it will also help to limit the pronation and supination of the foot, the cause of further problems for the runner.

Partial Sit-Up

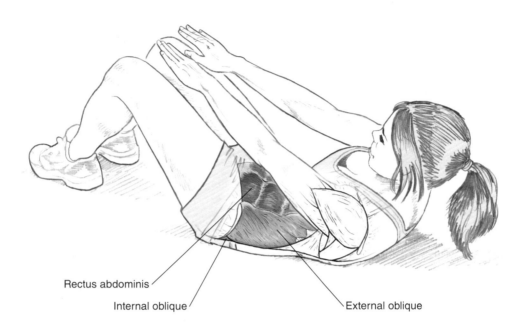

Rectus abdominis

Internal oblique

External oblique

Execution

1. Lie on a firm, supportive surface on your back with both knees bent and feet flat on floor. Have the hands resting loosely on or hovering slightly above the thighs.

2. Lift the arms a couple of inches and slowly raise the head and shoulders off the floor. Reach with both hands toward the knees and attempt to hold the position for 10 seconds. Repeat five times. Concentrate on performing the exercise smoothly without jerking; just as important, also ensure a slow return to the resting position between stretches.

Muscles Involved

Primary: rectus abdominis

Secondary: transversus abdominis, external oblique, internal oblique

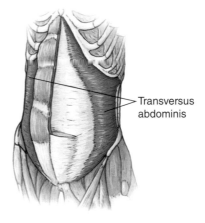

Transversus abdominis

Running Focus

It is impossible to overemphasize the importance of a stable core for a runner. Weak abdominal muscles cannot help support the back. If the torso crumples under the weight of the upper body, running becomes difficult and painful. This exercise also helps to preserve the link between the abdomen and the lower limbs, and it adds some strength to the knee lift, which in turn will enable the stride length to be maintained.

Seated Straight-Leg Extension

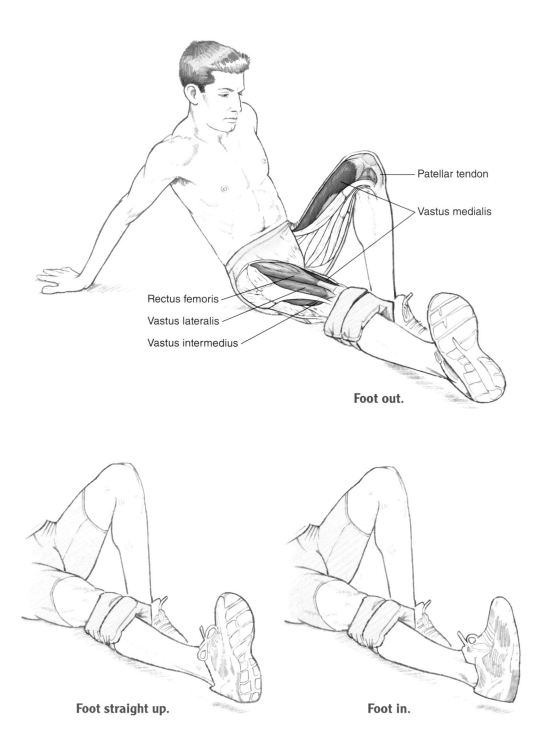

Patellar tendon

Vastus medialis

Rectus femoris

Vastus lateralis

Vastus intermedius

Foot out.

Foot straight up.

Foot in.

Execution

1. Sit on the floor with your arms behind you for support and one leg outstretched. In the early stages the ankles should not have weights attached, but as you become more adept, you may wish to attach up to 10 pounds of weight incrementally to improve strength.

2. Turn the foot outward and slowly lift the leg, locked straight but not hyperextended at the knee, until it is no more than six inches off the floor. Hold for 10 seconds, then, equally slowly, lower the ankle to the ground and rest. Repeat the exercise 10 times for 10 seconds and alternate with the opposite leg. The foot position can be changed to work all the muscles of the quadriceps evenly.

Muscles Involved

Primary: vastus medialis

Secondary: rectus femoris, vastus intermedius, vastus lateralis

Soft Tissue Involved

Primary: medial collateral ligament, patellar tendon

TECHNIQUE TIP
> ▸ **At first this may seem difficult, which is why you should not attach weights. The upper leg may well develop a tremor when first exercised in this fashion, but as strength is acquired, this will reduce and the whole exercise becomes easier.**

Running Focus

If sports medicine clinics banned runners with knee pain, they would become very lonely places! Unfortunately, too many coaches place far too much emphasis on general quadriceps development and fail to comprehend the role of the vastus medialis in stabilizing the knee and the prevention of patellofemoral pain. This is the most effective way of producing the increase in strength and power in this muscle to ward off the demon of anterior knee pain.

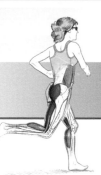

ANATOMY OF RUNNING FOOTWEAR

Runners who assiduously perform the strength-training regimen outlined in chapters 5 through 9 of this book, arrange their training to conform to the basic tenets of an intelligent training program as explained in chapter 2, and take the time to perform the injury-prevention exercises described in chapter 10 can still be stymied in their efforts to improve running performance. Simply by wearing the wrong training shoes or the wrong orthotic device for his or her foot type, a runner may short-circuit his or her well-intentioned efforts to improve. This chapter endeavors to present some sound wisdom about footwear and orthotic selection by presenting an overview of how and why running shoes are constructed for particular biomechanics and how runners can choose the right footwear and orthotics for their specific needs.

Why Wear Running Shoes?

Running shoes work for running because they are designed and manufactured to meet the demands of bearing three to four times the body's weight on impact, are designed for the biomechanics of running that are outlined in chapter 3, and are biomechanically (and, to a lesser extent, terrain) specific.

Running shoes are designed on lasts, or forms that are models of the human foot. These lasts have shapes ranging from curved to straight with variations on the degrees of the curve, which make the shoes appropriate for the various foot shapes of runners. The term *last* also applies to the methodology of construction. A combination-lasted shoe stitches the upper fabric underneath a cardboard heel to provide stability. A slip-lasted shoe stitches the upper directly to the midsole, ensuring flexibility. A full-board-last (cardboard from heel to toe) shoe is the most stable lasting technique but currently is almost nonexistent in shoe manufacturing.

Theoretically, curved slip-lasted shoes are designed for higher-arched, rigid feet, whereas straight combination-lasted shoes are designed for flatter, more flexible feet. Because flat feet tend to pronate (the inward rolling of the rear foot, controlled by the subtalar joint) more than high-arched feet, straight-lasted shoes, with the aid of stability devices embedded in the midsole, help limit the rate and amount of pronation. Conversely, runners who underpronate should wear curved to slightly curved slip-lasted shoes, which allow the foot to generate as much pronation as possible to help aid in shock absorption.

Many runners err in choosing shoes because they do not know what foot type they have. If an underpronator trains in stability shoes, predictable injuries like calf pain, Achilles tendinitis, and iliotibial band syndrome will occur. If an overpronator trains in a cushioning-only shoe, stress injuries (including fractures) to the foot, tibia, and the medial knee likely will occur. For most runners, a qualified employee at a running specialty store can evaluate foot biomechanics, possibly by using a treadmill and a video camera, and successfully recommend multiple shoe models that, in theory, will prevent injury and provide a pleasurable ride. Occasionally, evaluating the foot becomes tricky due to motion not seen clearly by the naked eye, and a slow-motion camera may be needed to ascertain true foot movement. This is rare and usually not found in recreational runners due to lower training volume and velocity. Understand that biomechanics can change; what was once corrected may no longer be a problem, and new problems can arise.

History of 20th-Century Running Shoes

The history of the running shoe in the 20th century begins with Spalding's introduction of the long-distance running shoe. The company outfitted the 1908 U.S. Olympic marathon team in its models, and based on observations of the marathon and the shoes' performances, it created a line of marathon shoes in 1909. Both high-top and low-top shoes with a pure gum sole and leather uppers were "full finished inside so as not to hurt the feet in a long race." Within five years, the gum rubber sole had been replaced by the leather sole, and the research and marketing of running shoes had begun in earnest, albeit in fits and starts.

Although Spalding continued tinkering with its running shoe models, the intrigue in running shoes sparked by the 1908 Olympic marathon in London gave way to a fascination with track spikes, particularly those manufactured by the Dassler brothers of Germany. Worn by Jesse Owens in the Munich Olympics, the spiked shoes were little more than a soft leather upper sewn to hard leather soles with permanent "nails" built into the soles to provide traction on the dirt tracks.

An interest in production of running shoes was rekindled in the United States in the mid-1960s through the mid-1970s, which ushered in the era of the running specialty business. Facing competition from the Japanese-imported Tiger running shoes, Hyde, New Balance, and Nike all began production of serious running shoes. The features of the new shoes were a higher heel, midsole cushioning material (EVA), and nylon uppers.

In some cases, the shoes were well made; in most cases, they were not. By the late 1970s, *Runner's World* began lab-testing the running shoes, and the manufacturers were forced to improve the quality of their shoes or lose market share. This change in the mind-set of the companies began a period of intense competition (that still lasts today) to provide the best fit with the most cushioning, stability, and durability in a shoe that looks good.

Components of Running Shoes

This section describes the components of the running shoe and their significance for the runner. The emphasis is on finding the right shoe, from a biomechanical and a fit standpoint. One part of the equation without the other could lead to injury. When purchasing shoes, remember that the cost of the shoe does not ensure its success. For one runner, an expensive shoe may only deplete his bank account without aiding performance; for another, the shoe may be expensive and perfect. Your foot type, shape, and biomechanics determine what is best when it comes to shoes.

Upper

The upper of a running shoe (figure 11.1) is the material that covers the top and the sides of the foot. It can be made of multiple pieces of fabric sewn or glue-welded together, or it can be made of a one-piece, seamless material. All current running shoes are of human-made materials (nylons) for breathability, comfort, and weight reduction. Leather is no longer used because of its lack of breathability, nonconforming shape after repeated use, weight, and cost.

The front of the upper is referred to as the *toe box* of the shoe (figure 11.2). It takes its shape from the last of the shoe (the form the shoe is built on), but its style is determined by the shoe designer to meet the needs of the shoe wearer. The toe boxes of many of the shoes built recently are wider and deeper to accommodate the higher-volume feet that seem to have become more prevalent as the second running boom has corralled more recreational

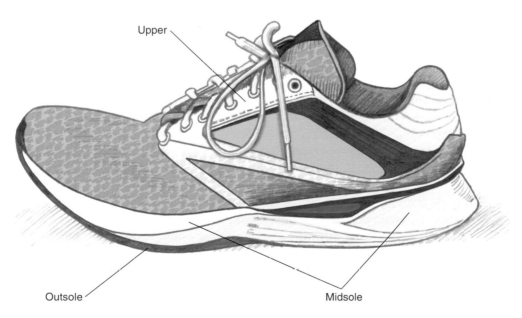

Figure 11.1 Lateral view of shoe: upper, midsole, and outsole.

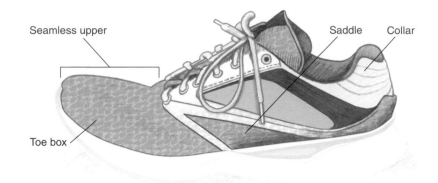

Seamless upper
Saddle Collar
Toe box

Figure 11.2 Upper.

runners with larger frames into the sport. The midfoot of the shoe's upper can be designed in conjunction with or independently of the lacing system (e.g., ghillie lacing) to allow for various upper fits. Occasionally, companies will attempt a nonsymmetrical lacing pattern ostensibly designed to improve the fit of the upper and remove "hot spots" (pre-blister-forming areas) from developing on the foot during running.

The design of the upper of the shoe determines the fit of the shoe—not the length of the shoe, but how the shoe envelops the foot. This is important because if the shoe fit is improper, the biomechanical needs of the runner may not be met. Only when the fit of the shoe is spot-on can the function (be it stability, motion control, or cushioning) work as designed. For example, if the fit of the upper is too baggy in the midfoot, excessive pronation can occur despite the presence of a medial support. The lack of a proper fit renders the stability device ineffective in combating the pronation it was designed to limit. Injuries can occur—in this case, tibial pain—even if a runner wears a shoe that is the correct category for his or her foot type.

This scenario often leads to disenchantment when purchasing shoes because of the confusion resulting from following the suggestions and guidelines and still not getting relief from pain. Here is a general point when purchasing shoes: If the shoe doesn't fit your foot well, it isn't the best shoe for you, regardless of whether its biomechanics are matched to your foot type. For example, it could be argued that for a mild overpronator, a cushioned shoe that fits perfectly is more stable than a mild stability shoe that is too roomy.

In conjunction with proper fit, a heel counter embedded in the upper material ensures a secure, mildly stable ride when running. Heel counters (figure 11.3) are hard plastic devices that stabilize the rear foot, helping the foot through the normal cycle of heel strike, midfoot stance (avoiding excess pronation), forefoot supination (the outward rolling of the forefoot), and toe-off from the smaller toes of the foot. Heel counters can be removed in shoes manufactured for underpronators, but the possibility of Achilles tendinitis is increased because of the increased movement of the calcaneus and the subsequent pulling on the Achilles tendon.

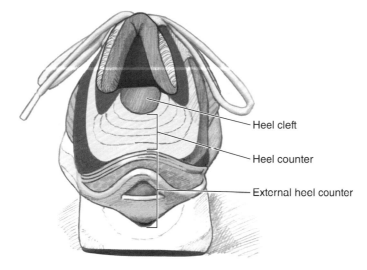

Figure 11.3 Heel counters and heel clefts.

Midsole

The midsole of a running shoe (figure 11.4) is made of EVA (ethylene vinyl acetate) or rubberized EVA used to cushion or stabilize the ride of the shoe during foot strike. Developed in the early 1970s as a cushioning material to rival polyurethane (which is denser and heavier), EVA has been combined with other proprietary cushioning materials such as air and gel as well as engineering designs like wave plates, footbridges, cantilevers, and truss systems to minimize impact shock generated during the foot strike and to guide the foot through its normal path.

The holy grail of midsole technology has been to find a material that provides a moderately soft ride and has the durability to withstand compression, which limits the life span of the shoe. A reasonable expectation for a running shoe's

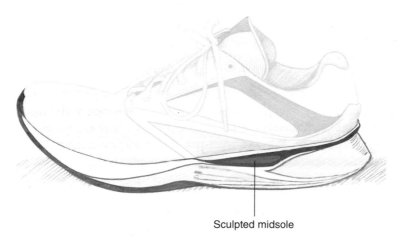

Sculpted midsole

Figure 11.4 Midsole.

life is 350 to 500 miles. The development of a midsole that could provide 750 miles of consistently comfortable running would be a boon both to runners and to the manufacturing company that patented the material.

The current crop of rubberized midsoles provide dramatically better cushioning than their "sheet" EVA predecessors from the 1970s, but there is an environmental cost associated with producing the material. Traditional EVA midsoles take approximately 1,000 years to entirely biodegrade. Some running shoe manufacturers are marketing eco-friendly "green" midsoles that are touted as environmentally sound because they degrade 50 times faster in a traditional landfill environment.

Most runners look at the outsoles of their shoes to determine whether the shoes need to be replaced. Unfortunately, when the outsole of a running shoe has worn away enough to show significant wear, the midsole has been long compromised in providing cushioning. Because midsoles provide cushioning, they also absorb and dampen the shock of impact. During a 30-minute run, each shoe lands on the ground approximately 2,700 times. That is multiplied by an impact force of three to four times a runner's body weight, so it's amazing that no more than a two-inch-thick wedge of EVA can withstand approximately 150 of these training runs before being replaced.

The midsole is also the part of the shoe that contains the various stability devices designed to prevent pronation. These devices are always placed on the medial side of the shoe, usually between the arch and the heel. The devices are located in this area to counter the effects of pronation, which is mainly controlled by the subtalar joint that is located in the area of the foot closest to this part of the shoe. Occasionally a shoe will be produced with forefoot posting (to prevent late-stage pronation of the forefoot), but this is a nontraditional method of design. Posting of the lateral side of the shoe is never done because increasing the rate and degree of pronation is problematic for pronators (leading to increased tibia discomfort) and needless for underpronators (a cushioned shoe allows for the foot to pronate as it needs to).

Outsole

The outsole of a running shoe (figure 11.5) has evolved dramatically from a materials standpoint from the gum rubber of the 1908 Spalding marathon trainers. The outsole (the part of the shoe that actually touches the road) is made of carbon and blown rubber composites used jointly to make for a durable yet appropriately flexible ride. Most runners strike the lateral heel of the foot upon impact. Hence, manufacturers place the most durable carbon rubber in this area of the shoe to ensure longevity of the outsole. Despite the added durability of the carbon rubber, excessive wear will still appear in that area of the shoe for most runners. This is to be expected and does not indicate a proclivity toward overpronation or underpronation. It simply means the runner is a heel striker.

If the outsole is completely worn through in the forefoot of the shoe, the midsole cushioning was compromised long before, and the shoe is worthless as a shock-absorbing entity. Because the outsole of the shoe lasts much

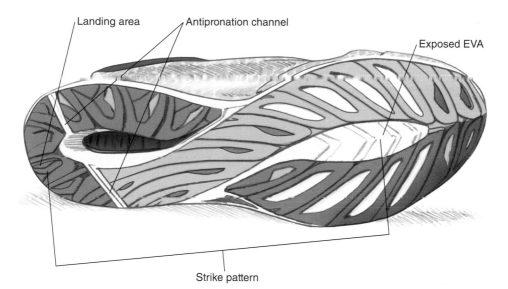

Landing area   Antipronation channel   Exposed EVA

Strike pattern

Figure 11.5   Outsole.

longer than the midsole cushioning, using outsole wear as a guide for when to replace your running shoes is erroneous. The best method of measuring the life of a shoe requires little work. Pay attention to the mileage on your shoes by keeping a log or quick estimation of miles per week multiplied by weeks of training, and after approximately 350 miles, replace your shoes when you begin to have aches or pains in your legs that you did not have for the first 350 miles of the shoe's life. Normally, if a shoe model is not correct for a runner's biomechanics, weight, flexibility, or foot shape (all factors that determine the best shoe), discomfort or injury will occur within the first 100 miles of running. Thus, the wrong shoe should rarely be confused with an old shoe.

Shoe manufacturers are constantly altering the strike path of a shoe's outsole and the surface pattern of the rubber to improve comfort and durability. Although these aims of the manufacturers seem to be worthwhile, the role of aesthetics in shoe design cannot be ignored. At every phase of design and development, the aesthetics of the shoe, its attractiveness to the consumer, must be weighed against the practicality of building the shoe and the effectiveness of the shoe for running purposes. Often the aesthetics of the shoe take precedence, and a much-hyped shoe proves to be a performance dud—albeit a dud with an expensive advertising campaign.

Insoles and Orthotics

Runners want to wear comfortable running shoes that help prevent injuries; however, because running shoes are not custom-made, there will always be a bit of a compromise when it comes to fit. Because each runner's foot is unique and not even symmetrical with the other foot, it becomes apparent that accommodations may be needed in order to enhance a running shoe's fit and its function. To customize the fit and function of their shoes, runners turn to insoles and orthotics.

Each pair of running shoes comes with an insole. It is made of EVA or a material combined with EVA to add comfort (shock absorption) and to aid the fit of the shoe. It costs less than 50 cents to manufacture, and it is mostly useless. It is removable, and for a good reason. Most runners remove the inexpensive insole and replace it with a more cushioned or more stable insole that actually has some resemblance to the shape of the human foot. In the past decade, over-the-counter replacement insoles have become a serious revenue generator for running specialty stores. The proliferation of these stores has led to more retail outlets for the sales of insoles, and the insole manufacturers have responded by producing good-quality products for less than $30.

It seems a bit redundant to spend $90 on a pair of shoes and $30 on a pair of insoles when you could just buy a $120 pair of running shoes. The true value of the insole is that it customizes the shoe to the runner's foot. Thus, the $90 shoe feels closer to a perfect fit than the $120 shoe because it more closely resembles a shoe made from a mold of the runner's own foot. Not only does the insole aid fit, but current insoles also help correct for poor biomechanics. They can be posted to compensate for pronation factors or high-arched to help prevent plantar fasciitis. They do work well, but they are not for every runner. Many runners can do without insoles because they do not have major biomechanical problems that their training will exacerbate. For those runners who have run a lot of miles in their lives, are training at a high volume, or have chronic injuries, insoles are a viable option. For those runners who do not find relief with an over-the-counter insole, the next step is to visit an expert (certified pedorthist or podiatrist) to obtain custom-made orthotics.

An orthotic device is meant to correct an anatomical or biomechanical abnormality. In theory, an orthotic device realigns the foot strike, which, in turn, alleviates any imbalances or weaknesses through the kinetic chain of events initiated by running. Do orthotics work? Sometimes.

Upon visiting a podiatrist or certified pedorthist, a runner should expect the following procedure to occur before an orthotic device is produced. The specialist should take a thorough history of running injuries, shoes worn, and remedies attempted. Measurements of leg length and an evaluation of joint mobility should be completed. X-rays can be taken, but they are often not necessary.

After evaluating the feet, the specialist will proceed to make plaster molds of them. The doctor will place each foot in a "neutral" position and wrap plaster-soaked strips of gauze around each one. The most important step is placing the foot in the neutral position. This position is the key element in producing an orthotic that works well. Because the goal of an orthotic is to correct, the foot must be in the neutral position so a cast can be fabricated that shows any corrections to be made. The difference between the runner's foot and the appropriate position of the runner's foot when in neutral is the correction that needs to be made. When the cast is sent to an orthotics lab to produce the orthotic, a technician will evaluate the cast and take more measurements. From the "negative" cast, a "positive" model is created from plaster and is ground to the specifications provided by the doctor.

A hard orthotic is fabricated from thermoplastic and filled with cushioning material. It is posted medially no more than 4 degrees to help position the foot in neutral at midstance. It is covered by a thin layer of synthetic material. A soft orthotic, also referred to as an accommodative orthotic, is more of a custom-made arch support than a posted orthotic. Its goal is less medial stabilization for pronation and more arch support for a runner with high, rigid arches.

Normally, a running orthotic will be full length, replacing the insole of the shoe. It is not uncommon for a laboratory to offer a three-quarter-length orthotic. Because most rear-foot motion issues can be alleviated with a three-quarter-length orthotic, logic would dictate that the weight-saving inherent to a three-quarter-length orthotic would be welcome. Unfortunately, the lack of a continuous surface under the complete length of the foot leads runners to fabricate their own system of completing the orthotic. Purchase an orthotic with a full-length cover.

The litmus test of a well-constructed orthotic is twofold. Does it fit comfortably into a running shoe (although it may be a different, larger shoe than you were wearing), and does the orthotic device eliminate the running injuries it was created to combat without causing other injuries? The answer should be a resounding yes! If not, contact your doctor for a follow-up appointment to reevaluate the orthotic.

The pairing of an orthotic device and a running shoe is a combination of art and science. If a hard, corrective orthotic is worn, a neutral cushioned shoe that encompasses the orthotic well and provides a good fit may suffice in eliminating any overpronation injuries. If a stability shoe is still needed with a hard, corrective orthotic, take caution to avoid the possibility of overposting the foot. This marriage of a stability shoe and corrective orthotic is a possible recipe for iliotibial band syndrome, an injury usually associated with under-pronators who stay on the lateral aspect of their foot through the foot strike, creating tightness in all the muscles and soft tissue laterally from the foot to the hip. At the first sign of pain on the lateral side of the knee or tightness in the hip area, reconsider the use of a stability shoe and corrective orthotic.

Underpronators who wear accommodative orthotics should continue to wear cushioned shoes. The only caveat, and this is true for overpronators with orthotics as well, is that an extra half size may be needed in order to fit the orthotic into a running shoe. The orthotic replaces the insole that comes with the shoe, but it is higher in volume and thus needs to be fit properly so that the biomechanics it is meant to promote during running can proceed seamlessly.

Barefoot Running

Barefoot running could have been included in chapter 9's list of exercises to strengthen the foot because that is essentially what barefoot running does best (along with developing some proprioceptive awareness). But daily barefoot training is not really a substitute for running in shoes. Given that most runners log the majority of their miles on asphalt, concrete, treadmills, and gravel-strewn trails, running barefoot daily seems a bit painful at the least; however, running without shoes does have many practical applications when used as a supplement to running training, much like the strength-training exercises outlined in chapters 5 and 6 of this book. It should not replace traditional (with shoes) training. The argument has been made that many African runners have trained barefoot and have had success (native South African Zola Budd is a famous example), but the counterargument is that all the world records are held by shoe-wearing runners.

Proponents of barefoot running tout the muscular strength gained through barefoot running, which is an accurate assessment in the proper context. Advocates of barefoot running also tout the psychological release derived from running on sand and lush grass, which may also be because sand and lush grass are normally found in places more likely to be idyllic, although it is a tenuous connection to aiding running performance.

The best reason to do some barefoot running on lush grass or hard-packed sand (not more than twice a week and no more than 100 meters straight for a total of 400 meters per session to begin) is to train the muscles of your feet to work differently than they do when running shoes are worn. Barefoot running forces the feet to work, preventing atrophy in the muscles of the foot that function the same way during every run in running shoes with or without orthotics. The antiorthotic movement in running espouses mixing in barefoot running and running in neutral shoes for overpronators to force the foot to strengthen itself to prevent future injuries. Just as the exercises in this book have detailed how to strengthen your body to improve running performance, barefoot running can help strengthen your feet to withstand the countless training miles required of them. As with all strength training, if you feel pain while barefoot running, stop.

Summary

The ultimate goal of a well-designed and constructed running shoe and orthotic device is to promote injury-free and comfortable running. Extra cushioning to limit the impact forces of the foot strike, stability devices adding medial posting to limit pronation generated by the subtalar joint, and transitional EVA densities to ease the transition from heel strike to midstance are all designed to meet this goal. Appropriate footwear and orthotic devices (matched to a runner's biomechanical needs), when combined with the strength-training program for the lower leg and foot presented in chapter 9, should eliminate all leg and foot injuries. One caveat is that the running shoe and orthotic must be appropriate to the foot that wears it, and the shoe and orthotic device must be replaced when its cushioning, stability, and accommodative properties are compromised. Normally, a running shoe can be expected to last at least 350 miles, an aftermarket insole should last through every other shoe purchase, and a custom orthotic should last at least two years (although the cover may need to be replaced).

Trained employees at running specialty stores can help runners match current running shoes with the appropriate foot types and match feet with nonprescription insoles that provide similar protection as orthotic devices, but are not custom-made by a podiatrist.

The effectiveness of any running shoe and orthotic device hinges not just on biomechanics but also on fit. A well-constructed shoe that is the right biomechanical choice for a runner may not function correctly if the shoe is ill-fitted to the foot. When purchasing a shoe, make sure the shoe is neither too long or too short, nor too wide or too narrow. Also, try the new shoes with the orthotic device to be worn in order to replicate the fit of the shoe-and-insert combination. Remember, if it doesn't work in the store, it is not going to work on the road, trail, or track!

Chapters 5 through 9 of this book deal with strength training and the specific anatomy affected by properly performed resistance exercises. This chapter deals with alternative forms of exercise that complement the strength-training exercises detailed in the previous chapters. Specifically, this chapter examines water running and plyometrics as performance-enhancing training tools for runners.

Full-body conditioning is an important training element because it can diminish the injury potential that a repetitive, high-impact exercise such as running can have on the musculoskeletal system. By substituting a deep-water running session for a land running session, you can avoid countless tons of force on the body's anatomy without a concurrent loss in cardiovascular stimulation. Also, incorporating plyometrics into a training plan strengthens muscles, aiding the ability to withstand the impact of accumulated running training miles. It also helps in recovery from injury (when performed at the appropriate time), and it can improve running economy.

Water Running

Most runners have been introduced to water running as a rehabilitative tool for maintaining cardiorespiratory fitness after incurring an injury that precludes dryland running. However, runners should not assume that aquatic training's only benefit is injury rehabilitation. Running in water, specifically deep-water running (DWR), is a great tool for preventing overuse injuries associated with a heavy volume of aerobic running training. Also, because of the drag associated with running in water, an element of resistance training is associated with water running that does not exist in traditional running-based training.

Although shallow-water running is a viable alternative to DWR, its benefits tend to be related to form and power. Although the improvement of form and power is important, it comes at a cost. Because shallow-water running requires impact with the bottom of a pool, it has an impact component (although the force is mitigated by the density of the water). For a runner rehabbing a lower leg injury, shallow-water running could pose a risk of injury. More important, balance and form are easier to attain in shallow-water running because of a true foot plant. Fewer core muscles are engaged to center the body, as in DWR, and there is a resting period during contact that does not exist in DWR. For our purposes, all water-related training exercises focus on DWR.

In performing a DWR workout, proper body positioning is important (figure 12.1). The depth of the water should be sufficient to cover the entire body: Only the tops of the shoulders, the neck, and the head should be above the surface of the water. The feet should not touch the bottom of the pool. Runners tend to have more lean body mass than swimmers, making them less buoyant; therefore, a flotation device will be necessary. If a flotation device is not worn, body position can become compromised and an undue emphasis is placed on the muscles of the upper body and arms to keep the body afloat.

Once buoyed in the water, assume a body position similar to dryland running. Specifically, the head is centered, there is a slight lean forward at the waist, and the chest is "proud," or expanded, with the shoulders pulled back, not rotated forward. Elbows are bent at 90 degrees, and movement of the arms is driven by the shoulders. The wrists are held in a neutral position, and the hands, although not clenched, are more closed than on dry land in order to

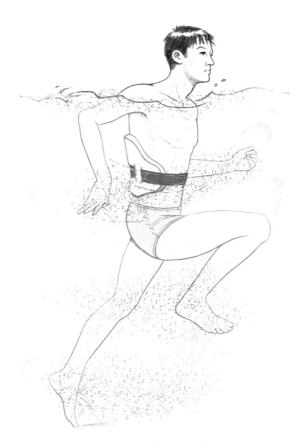

Figure 12.1   Proper body position for deep-water running.

push through the resistance of the water. (See figure 12.2 for an example of poor body position during DWR.) The strength gained from performing wrist curls and reverse wrist curls (see chapter 6) are beneficial for this.

Leg action is more akin to faster-paced running than general aerobic running because of the propulsive force needed for overcoming the resistance caused by the density of the water. The knee should be driven upward to an approximate 75-degree angle at the hip. The leg is then driven down to almost full extension (avoiding hyperextension) before being pulled upward directly under the buttocks before the process is repeated with the other leg.

During the gait cycle, the feet change position from no flexion (imagine standing on a flat surface) when the knee is driving upward to approximately 65 degrees of plantarflexion (toes down) at full extension. This foot movement against resistance both facilitates the mechanics of running form and promotes joint stability and muscle strength as a result of overcoming the resistance caused by drag.

Due to the unnatural training environment (water) and the resistance created when driving the arms and legs, improper form is common when beginning a DWR training program. Specifically, it is common to make a punting-like motion with the forward leg instead of snapping it down as shown in the B motion on page 24. This error is due to fatigue of the hamstrings from the water resistance, resulting in poor mechanics. To correct this error, rest at the onset of the fatigue, and don't perform another repetition until the time goal is met. Do not try to push through it. You won't gain fitness, and you will gain poor form.

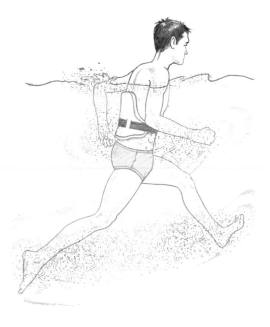

Figure 12.2   Incorrect body position for deep-water running.

Figure 12.3 shows a DWR technique that most closely resembles dryland running form. It is the best technique for facilitating proper running form while training in deep water. A high-knee alternative does exist (figure 12.4), but it is less effective in mimicking the nuances of proper running form. Instead, it more closely resembles the form used on a stair-stepping exercise machine. There is little running action other than the lift phase and therefore very little muscle involvement.

DWR is effective because it elevates the heart rate, similar to dryland running. And because of the physics of drag, it requires more muscular involvement, thus strengthening more muscles than dryland running does without the corresponding overuse injuries associated with such training. Specifically, it eliminates the thousands of impact-producing foot strikes incurred during non-DWR running.

DWR is easily integrated into a running training program either as a substitute for an aerobic run, lactate, or $\dot{V}O_2$max effort or as a supplemental workout, such as a second running workout of the day. Because pace is easily controlled

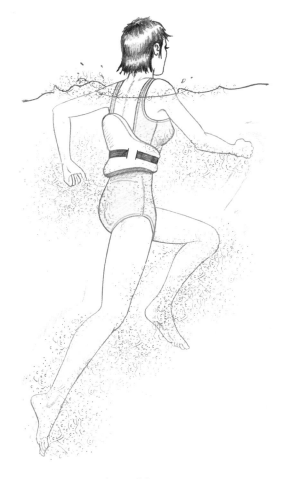

Figure 12.3   Deep-water running, traditional form.

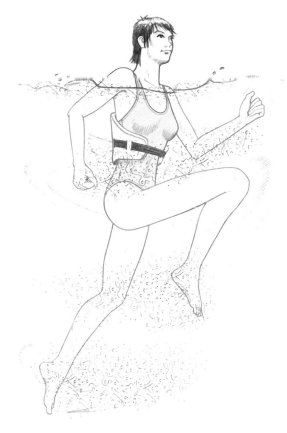

Figure 12.4   Deep-water running, high-knee form.

by speeding up or slowing down leg turnover, adjusting efforts based on heart rate or perceived effort is simple. Studies have found that heart rates during water running are about 10 percent lower than during land running, so a heart rate of 150 beats per minute (bpm) during water running equates to a heart rate of 165 bpm on land. Also, perceived effort is greater in water because of the combination of greater muscle involvement and the warmer temperatures of most pools. Because running for an hour in the pool is boring to most runners, we recommend 50 minutes in a pool as a good substitute for an on-land easy run; fartlek and interval-type efforts should be the emphasis of DWR training. Also, multiple intense efforts akin to speed work on land can be performed weekly because of the lack of ground impact. The following are two sample DWR workouts.

Sample Lactate Workout

The goal of this workout is to elevate the blood-lactate accumulation. At the end of each subsequent repetition, muscle fatigue should be increasingly present because the one-minute rest does not allow full recovery. This is not an easy workout, but it would not be a true speed session.

Warm-up: 15 min easy running + 4 × :30 @ 5K race pace (perceived effort)

2 × 10 min @ 10K race pace (perceived effort) with 1 min recovery jog

1 × 15 min @ 10K race pace (perceived effort) with 1 min recovery jog

Cool-down: 10 min easy running

Sample $\dot{V}O_2$max Workout

The goal of this workout is to simulate 5K race effort. Because pace can't be replicated in a pool, the emphasis of the workout is on perceived effort. Heart rate can be used; if you know your training zones from an LT test and you own a waterproof heart rate monitor, the exact effort can be substituted. Rest is given to allow for proper form on each repetition. Note that, as in running on dry land, body position is an important component of running efficiency. Good body position (as described and illustrated earlier in the chapter) leads to a more productive workout. This would be a moderately hard effort for a trained runner and a difficult effort for a beginner.

Warm-up: 15 min easy running + 4 × :30 @ 5K race pace (perceived effort)

5 × 2 min @ 5K race pace (perceived effort) with 2 min recovery jog

3 × 3 min @ 5K race pace (perceived effort) with 3 min recovery jog

3 × 2 min @ 5K race pace (perceived effort) with 2 min recovery jog

Cool-down: 10 min easy running

Plyometrics

The term *plyometrics* is mysterious to many distance runners, although it is a common training tool for many elite distance runners, middle-distance runners, and sprinters, most professional athletes, and many athletes rehabilitating from injuries. For the noninitiated, it sounds like, and at times is represented as, a hyperspeed method of improving performance. Just perform plyometrics, drink amino acid–laced recovery drinks, and voilà, instant performance improvements.

By definition, *plyometrics* means measurable increases, in this case through body-weight exercises. Because it is the *use* of strength, not raw strength, that contributes to speed development, plyometric exercises have one main goal: the conversion of strength to speed by generating a large amount of force quickly. Plyometric exercises train the neurological and muscular systems to increase the speed at which the body's strength can be used. By performing plyometric exercises, runners can measurably improve running performance, but not in the way they may think.

A by-product of the development of muscular power is an improvement in running economy. Running economy is the cost, or amount of oxygen, required to maintain a defined pace. The less oxygen used to maintain a certain pace relative to other runners or your previous measurement, the better the running economy. It does not quantify the efficiency of running form (the terms are often confused), although running form may affect running economy.

Plyometric exercises trigger improved running economy through recruitment of muscle fibers in a way that distance training does not. A plyometrically trained athlete's muscle contractions are shorter in duration; because less strength is required to perform the contraction (a result of both increased strength and neurological development), running economy improves. This chain of events leads to faster performances caused by the delay of muscle fatigue.

But, unlike DWR, plyometrics cannot be substituted for running training to improve performance for distance runners. Although DWR has an impact on LT and $\dot{V}O_2$max, plyometric exercises train the neuromuscular systems with almost no impact on the cardiothoracic systems described in chapter 2. Without running training, plyometric training could not sustain improvements in running performance.

There is debate about the phase of training in which plyometrics should be incorporated. There are no definitive answers, but we suggest one plyometric session per week during lactate training and two sessions per week during $\dot{V}O_2$max training. The workout should be done before the LT or $\dot{V}O_2$max workout takes place, in a separate training session if possible, and not on recovery days.

The plyometric workout should be sufficient in duration to develop muscular fatigue, but not so difficult that the running workout is compromised. The neurological component of the workout is as important as the muscular strength derived from exercises, so performing the exercises to exhaustion can overload the muscles for the workout to follow and performance improvement could be hindered.

Following are four beginning plyometric exercises that can be incorporated into a running program. The exercises do not all meet the true definition of a plyometric exercise (eccentric muscle contraction, inertia, concentric contraction), but because they do involve explosive muscle-contraction movements, most current training programs include them as plyometric drills. These can be performed all in one session, as one set only, as multiple (two or three) sets of each for a heavier day, or as just one or two exercises with a single set for an easy preworkout. Limit the total number of repetitions or touches to no more than eight per exercise (except for box steps, which can be done in one-minute intervals at varying speeds) and the total number of sets to no more than five per exercise.

The number of exercises performed and the number of reps or touches are dependent on many factors: The familiarity of the runner with plyometric exercises, the difficulty of the workout to be performed after the plyometric session, and the runner's fitness. Following the exercises are some guidelines for performance.

Frogger

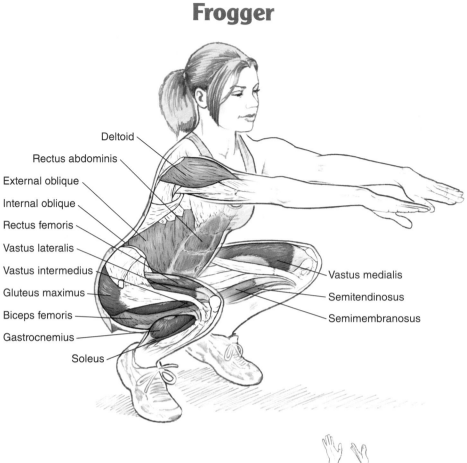

Deltoid
Rectus abdominis
External oblique
Internal oblique
Rectus femoris
Vastus lateralis
Vastus intermedius
Gluteus maximus
Biceps femoris
Gastrocnemius
Soleus

Vastus medialis
Semitendinosus
Semimembranosus

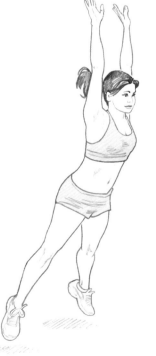

Midair position.

Execution

1. Position the body in a full squat position with feet slightly apart. The thighs are horizontal to the ground with the lower back gently arched. The head is centered and the chin is slightly raised. Arms are extended in front of the body.

2. Inhale deeply while sweeping the arms backward and then quickly forward, developing momentum for the legs to explode from the full squat position at a 60-degree angle, throwing the arms above the head. Upon reaching the apex of the jump, prepare to land, and lower the body into the same body position (full squat) as when the exercise started.

3. Upon landing and reestablishing proper squat form, immediately repeat the jump.

Muscles Involved

Primary: quadriceps, gluteus maximus, gastrocnemius, soleus

Secondary: hamstrings, deltoid, rectus abdominis, external oblique, internal oblique

Running Focus

The frogger is a propulsive exercise that requires the athlete to explode from the start position, engaging the quadriceps, hamstrings, and glutes. Although it has a very practical application for sprinters (the improvement of the starting motion from a block), the frogger, like all plyometric exercises, can also aid the distance runner by increasing running economy by strengthening the impacted muscles, leading to less energy consumption during distance running.

A-Step Depth Jump

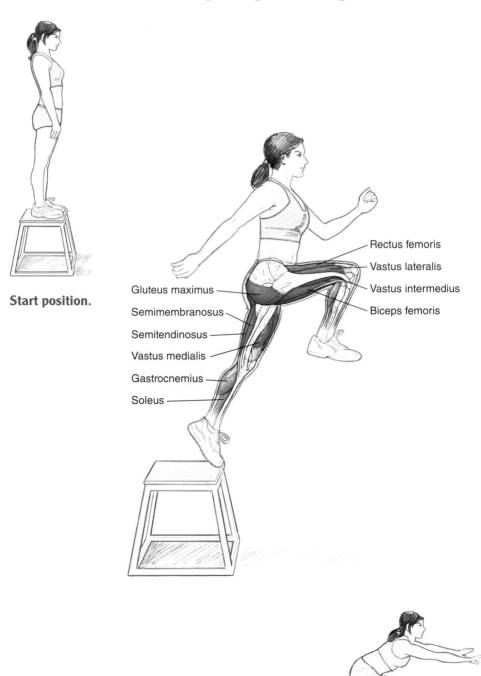

Start position.

Rectus femoris

Vastus lateralis

Vastus intermedius

Biceps femoris

Gluteus maximus

Semimembranosus

Semitendinosus

Vastus medialis

Gastrocnemius

Soleus

Landing position.

Execution

1. Standing on a platform, step forward using the knee action of the A motion of running from chapter 3.
2. Land on both feet and, reacting as quickly as possible, spring immediately back up into the air in a frogger-like fashion.
3. Maintain a neutral posture and a balanced, elevated chest position throughout the exercise. Do not attempt to absorb the landing on impact; rather, react as quickly and as fast as possible, even if this sacrifices height gained.

Muscles Involved

Primary: quadriceps, gluteus maximus, hamstrings

Secondary: gastrocnemius, soleus

TECHNIQUE TIP

▶ **Use the arms to add to the speed by drawing them back before stepping off the platform and swinging them vigorously upward as the feet hit the ground. Keep the back in neutral alignment, not arched or rounded.**

Running Focus

This involves an eccentric contraction, stepping down from the box, leading into a concentric contraction, a traditional plyometric drill with the added bonus of beginning the exercise with a running-specific A step.

Box Step-Up

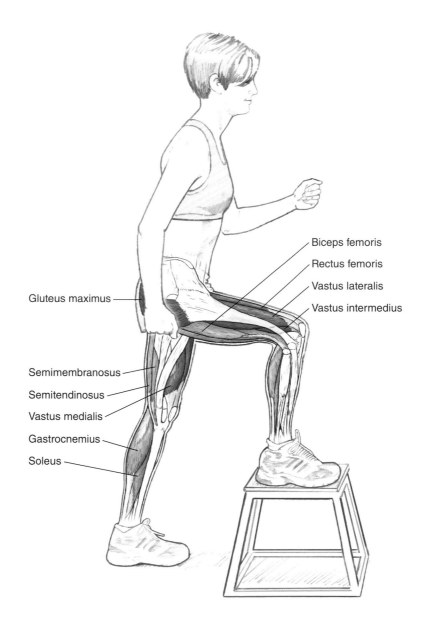

Biceps femoris

Rectus femoris

Vastus lateralis

Vastus intermedius

Gluteus maximus

Semimembranosus

Semitendinosus

Vastus medialis

Gastrocnemius

Soleus

Execution

1. Stand with good posture facing a plyometric box or weight bench. The height of the box should not be higher than the knee.

2. Engage the quadriceps on one side, lift that foot off the ground, and place it on the bench at a 90-degree angle at the knee. Step up with the other leg in the same manner so that you are standing on the box or bench.

3. Immediately step down, reversing the pattern used to step up.

Muscles Involved

Primary: quadriceps, gluteus maximus

Secondary: hamstrings, gastrocnemius, soleus

Running Focus

This exercise mimics the A motion presented in chapter 3; however, it has little impact, and can be performed for significantly longer. Instead of touches, this exercise can be measured in minutes; for example, a sample workout could be 2 × 1 minute of slow step-ups followed by 2 × 1 minute of fast step-ups, followed by 2 × 1 minute of slow step-ups. Changing the speed of the step-up, the height of the platform stepped onto, and the time interval allows for variation. The exercise seems benign, but five minutes of stepping is plenty of time for a good burn of the glutes and quadriceps.

Cone Jump

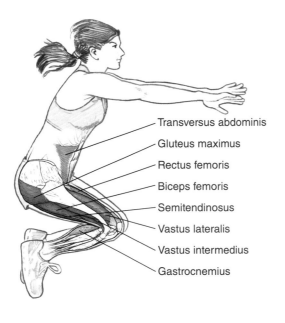

Transversus abdominis
Gluteus maximus
Rectus femoris
Biceps femoris
Semitendinosus
Vastus lateralis
Vastus intermedius
Gastrocnemius

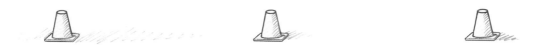

Execution

1. Place three or four cones two feet apart in a straight line.
2. Stand six inches behind the first cone in a partial squat position with the arms by the sides.
3. Driving the arms, explode forward in a modified frogger, landing in a slightly deeper squat than when starting. Repeat over each cone.

Muscles Involved

Primary: gluteus maximus, quadriceps, hamstrings

Secondary: gastrocnemius, transversus abdominis

TECHNIQUE TIP
▸ Pause only briefly upon landing. To perform a less explosive version of this exercise, keep your feet level with each other and parallel to the floor.

Running Focus

The eccentric contraction is the landing, and the concentric contraction is the takeoff. The quads extend during takeoff, and the hamstrings and glutes eccentrically contract when landing.

VARIATION

Lateral Cone Jump

This variation changes the muscles used to include the gluteus medius and minimus, which aid in abduction, and the adductor muscles. Perform the exercise by turning sideways at the start, so your side is facing the cones. Perform the jump with the same body position, just move sideways over the cones.

EXERCISE FINDER

MOTION

UPPER TORSO

ARMS AND SHOULDERS

CORE

UPPER LEGS

LOWER LEGS AND FEET

INJURY PREVENTION

FULL-BODY CONDITIONING

ABOUT THE AUTHORS

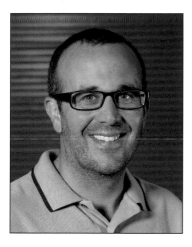

Joe Puleo is currently the head men's and women's cross-country and track and field coach at Rutgers University-Camden. He is also the head running coach for Cadence Cycling and MultiSport Center, a premiere training center in Philadelphia featured by the *New York Times*, *Outside, Men's Journal, Men's Health, Shape, GQ*, and *Triathlete Magazine.* His responsibilities as lead instructor include coaching the United States Marine Corps global running program.

His previous 20 years of experience include coaching multiple high school state champions in track and field, NCAA Division III All-Americans in the 100 meter, the 800 meter, and cross-country, male and female winners at the prestigious Penn Relays and NYRRC Marathon Tune-Up, and an Olympic Trials qualifier in the marathon. Puleo has also coached three World Championship teams for the United States Armed Forces, two marathon teams and a cross-country team.

Formerly a nationally ranked age-group triathlete, Mr. Puleo has competed in over 100 multisport events and over 300 cross-country, track, and road races in the past 24 years. Mr. Puleo lives in Phoenixville and Mt. Gretna, Pennsylvania, with his wife, Lyndi, and their three children.

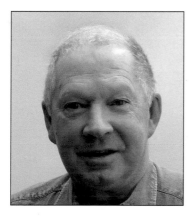

Patrick Milroy has been the Chief Medical Officer for the Road Runners Club since 1998. Previously, he was a medical advisor and contributor to *Runner's World Magazine* from 1991 to 2007. He was similarly involved with precursors *Jogging Magazine* and *Running Magazine.* While working at The Knoll, Dr. Milroy was also Chief Medical Officer and sole medical practitioner for the North Cheshire Sports Injuries Clinic from 1984 to 2002.

Dr. Milroy has received the award of Fellow twice (from the Institute of Sports Medicine in 1999 and from the UK Faculty of Sport and Exercise Medicine in 2006). He served as a medical officer for many athletic events, including the World Half Marathon Championships, Commonwealth Games, Team England Commonwealth Games (4 times), British Athletics Federation, and Great Britain Team at the World Junior Championships (3 times) and European Junior Championships (2 times).

Dr. Milroy is the author of *Sports Injuries,* coauthor of the *AAA Runner's Guide,* and author of numerous other articles on sport- and exercise-related topics for journals, magazines and newspapers. He is also an accomplished runner as winner of the World Medical Games 5000m and half marathon in 1980, 1982, and 1984 and winner of the European Medical Games 20K, 5K, and 1500m in 1983. His personal best in the marathon is 2 hours and 26 minutes.

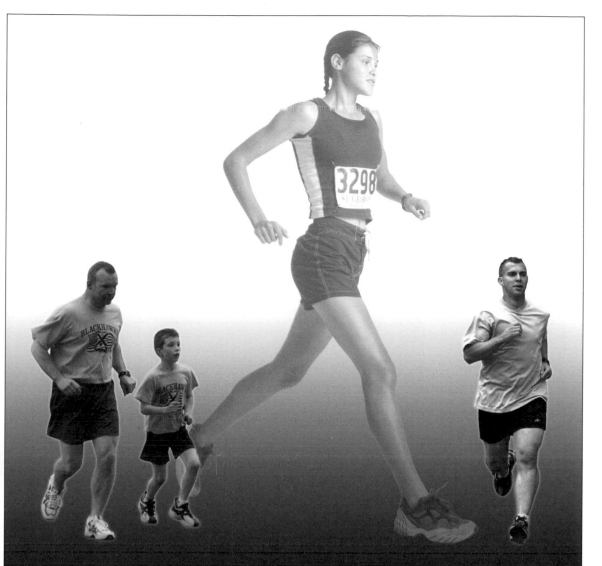
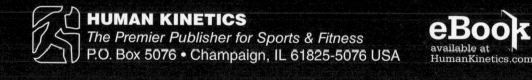

ANATOMY SERIES

Each book in the *Anatomy Series* provides detailed, full-color anatomical illustrations of the muscles in action and step-by-step instructions that detail perfect technique and form for each pose, exercise, movement, stretch, and stroke.

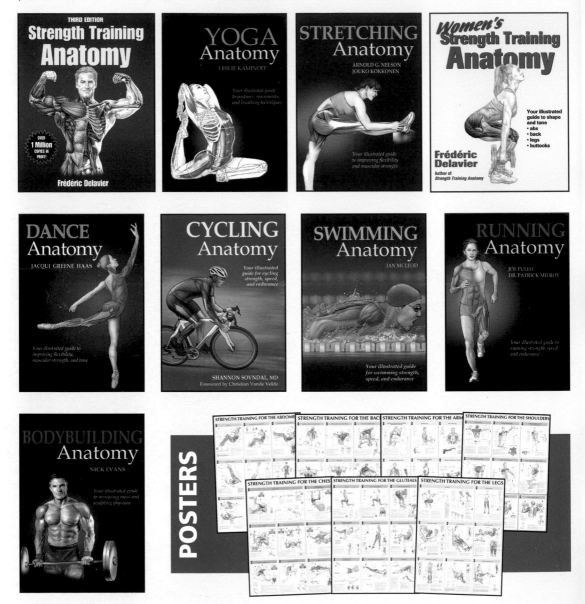

HUMAN KINETICS
The Premier Publisher for Sports & Fitness
P.O. Box 5076, Champaign, IL 61825-5076